"A DELIGHTFUL, DIRT-ROAD VERSION OF HERRIOT."
—*Birmingham News*

"Tells of the many trials and tribulations of a country animal doctor and the importance of diplomacy and a sense of humor . . . McCormack quickly becomes a master at both."
—*Kirkus Reviews*

"Captures the people and animals of southern Alabama and makes the reader care about them . . . Amusing and heart-tugging . . . Full of folksy wit and down-to-earth recollections."
—*The Chattanooga Free Press*

"Vibrant . . . Wonderfully reminiscent of the animal tales of James Herriot, only set in the Deep South."
—*The Nashville Banner*

"A collection of heartwarming, hilarious anecdotes."
—*The Choctaw Advocate*

Fields and Pastures New

Fields and Pastures New

MY FIRST YEAR AS A COUNTRY VET

Dr. John McCormack

FAWCETT COLUMBINE • NEW YORK

A Fawcett Columbine Book
Published by Ballantine Books

Copyright © 1995 by John McCormack
Excerpt from *A Friend of the Flock* copyright © 1997 by John McCormack

All rights reserved under International and Pan-American Copyright Conventions. Published in the United States by Ballantine Books, a division of Random House, Inc., New York, and simultaneously in Canada by Random House of Canada Limited, Toronto.

http://www.randomhouse.com

Library of Congress Catalog Card Number:97-90457

ISBN: 0-449-22536-4

This edition published by arrangement with Crown Publishers, Inc.

Cover design by Cathy Colbert
Cover photo © by Gerald French/FPG International
Cover photo insets *(left to right):* © Dave Gleiter/FPG International; ©Mike Barrett; © Ken Ross/ FPG International

Manufactured in the United States of America

First Ballantine Books Edition: November 1997

10 9 8 7 6 5 4 3 2 1

This book is dedicated to my family. It is for Jan, my wife and best friend, whose encouragement and enthusiasm have helped to create an exciting thirty-seven-year adventure and who instilled in me the grit to tackle the difficult and unknown. It is for my late parents, Martha and Edward, who gave me guidance and taught me the value of common sense. It is for Milton and Christine Smith, who have always believed in me, even when I took their only daughter to far-off Choctaw County. And for my children:

Tom and Mary
Lisa, Mike, and Christine Barrett
Paul, Kim, Dillon, and Maddox

They inspire me and serve to remind me of what is really important.

ACKNOWLEDGMENTS

FOR THEIR SUPPORT and assistance, I would like to thank the following people: Peggy Vaughn, Cindy Huff, Darlyne Llewellyn, Teresa McClure, Elizabeth Carroll, Kelli Barritt, and Brent Hix.

I would also like to give special thanks to Peter Ginna, Patrick Sheehan, and Elke Villa at Crown Publishers.

And a very special thanks to my friend and agent Ethan Ellenberg, whose phone call found me doctoring cows in a barn. I appreciate his faith, his encouragement, and his never letting me quit.

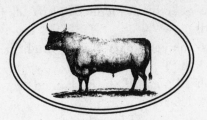

INTRODUCTION

I'M A VETERINARIAN, and I consider it an honor to be entrusted with the health care of animals. I enjoy most everything about my job except the name. So many people, including our own kin and friends, can't seem to get such a difficult word correct.

"Is this the venetian?" callers frequently inquire.

"Let me go to the window and look," is what I've always wanted to say but never had enough nerve. I reckon it does look kind of like the word "venetian" in the Yellow Pages.

"That doctor over in Meridian told me this here dog's got the heartworms," a pulpwood cutter said as he lifted his coonhound up onto the examination table. "But I wanted a second opinion from an out-of-town vegetarian." Say what?

It seems like we get called all sorts of names that start with the letter *V.* I've been called the veneer, veteran, vetran, vitnery, vanadium, vendetta, and even the Vatican.

Not long ago I met a lady at some sort of community gathering. When she found out what I did she was elated.

"Oh, my nephew really, really wants to be a venary. Do you think you could call somebody over at the vestibule school and ask them to let him in?"

Another nice lady whose twenty-year-old shepherd dog was very ill decided that we should call the "divinity school" for advice, where brilliant minds and higher authority figures were available.

There was certainly no doubt that the poor animal needed the benefit of divine intervention, not to mention a new set of kidneys, teeth, and joints. I carefully explained to the lady that folks at the divinity school were a whole lot better at shepherding to sick flocks than flocking to sick shepherds.

"Perhaps a call to the veterinary college might be more appropriate," I suggested.

"Oh yes, that's what I meant!" she exclaimed. "I was just so upset I got confused. I knew it started with a *V*."

But of all the *V* names that I have been called, my least favorite is "venereal." It just detracts from the public image that most of us in the profession are trying to create.

"I'm looking for John McCormack, Venereal," I heard the UPS guy say one morning while I was at the barbershop just up the hill from our place. "Got a package here for him."

Serious guffawing erupted from the regular crowd of early-morning sitters and liars at what should have been called the Clown and Comedy Haircut Shop. Of course those regulars had no problem with the proper pronunciation for the long and difficult word for animal doctor, since they knew everything.

"There he is, right over there," snickered Loren Caudle, my main man, best friend, golfing buddy, political consultant, and local pharmacist. "But you got it all wrong, he's not the venereal, he's the vetran. Ain't that right, vetran?" New guffawing erupted, even from the Baptist preacher getting clipped in the middle chair.

"Thanks a lot, farmist," I said sarcastically. "It's nice that you cleared that up for all of us."

By then the poor delivery man was really confused. He didn't know whether to drop the package and run or just join the parade of clowns. He did the former.

"What's in the package, venereal?" asked Harry, the head clown.

"Parvo vaccine, I imagine," I replied.

"Porno vaccine?" More peals of laughter, thigh slapping, and snorting erupted. There's no way to maintain your dignity at the Clown and Comedy Haircut Shop.

Not being called Doctor, or being called a "venereal" or a "vegetarian," is really only a minor irritation to most of us. As Carney Sam Jenkins, a self-taught colleague, dirt-road philosopher, and gifted seer used to say, "Doc, it don't matter what they call you, just as long as they call you!"

As the above might suggest, a sense of humor is an essential item for a veterinarian—ahead even of a pickup truck and close behind a tolerant spouse. I hope the episodes in this book will help to explain some of the joys, frustrations, surprises, and, especially, the comical experiences that nearly every veterinarian shares.

As a working veterinarian, I never thought of myself as an author. I didn't set out to write anything more than an occasional article on livestock health for a farm magazine or a description of a practical bovine surgical procedure for a veterinary journal. But then two things happened. First, I found that I actually enjoyed writing, and apparently others seemed to understand what I was trying to say on the printed page. They called and asked for more, and when a humorous article slipped out they even laughed, which surprised me. This led to a regular column in *Hoard's Dairyman* and irregular offerings in a local newspaper and a veterinary journal. Second, a new friend in the big city called a few times and encouraged me to write a more extended narrative about my experiences in the general practice of veterinary medicine.

This book is the end result of those phone calls. It tells about the first months of my family's venture into the practice of veterinary medicine in an Alabama county that had never before supported such an enterprise. My experiences might also be the experiences of my colleagues, many of whom could have written this book, but didn't. Perhaps they can't stand the thought of sitting down for hours and hours scribbling on a yellow legal pad and wondering whether their grammar and sentence structure are editorially acceptable. Or maybe, like so many things in a vet's life, they just haven't gotten around to it yet.

Perhaps the real reason I wrote this book is because I want people to know about veterinary medicine and how it was practiced in 1963. Many of the treatments have changed since that time, but the challenges and rewards have not. The animal owner–veterinarian bond can be very strong at times, yet very fragile and strained when things get crossed up. I am proud to say that my closest friendships, outside my family, have been with my clients. In these pages, I hope readers will get to know some of the workings of the small family farm and how these down-to-earth people confront their hardships and disappointments with so much good humor.

Fields and Pastures New

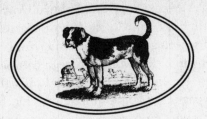

Chapter 1

AS I GUIDED the packed rental truck into Choctaw County, I had an unusual feeling that this was where I belonged. I wondered if Jan, my faithful wife and best friend following in the old station wagon, had the same sensation. I was sure that she was already happily making plans with four-year-old Tom and barely two-year-old Lisa for picnics and excursions through the new territory.

All our possessions were loaded on the truck and atop the station wagon. Mickey and Go Back, our Border collie and tabby cat, were riding shotgun with me, both snoozing, Mickey curled on the seat and Go Back atop the seat back. I was embarking on the goal and dream of nearly every veterinarian—his or her own private practice.

The autumn of 1963 had been a dreary, wet time in south Alabama, and this day in early November was following the pattern. Drizzling rain and forty-degree temperature is unpleasant to most Southerners, whether man or beast. I felt for the beef cattle alongside the road with their backs arched, their heads down, and eyes half closed, trudging barnward through the mud and into the chilly northwest wind.

The veterinary facts about cows and inclement weather stored away somewhere in my brain immediately sprang to mind and I quickly created a likely list of problems. Bronchitis, pneumonia, calf diphtheria, down cows, and weak calves were all problems that I could expect to see in the weeks to come.

We were ready to build a practice from the ground up the way we wanted it, with all the rewards of having done it by ourselves. We were also blissfully ignorant of some of the problems that stood in our way.

I had earned a D.V.M. degree from Auburn University in 1960 and had worked part-time for Dr. Chuck Otto in east Alabama while in school. Then I had served a three-month internship in his busy mixed practice when my formal classwork had been completed.

After graduation, I spent nine months in Louisiana, working as an inspector at a meatpacking plant and handling Dr. Bob Taylor's practice while he and his wife enjoyed an extended tour of Europe.

My next tour of duty was with Dr. Max Foreman in Foley, Alabama, near the Gulf of Mexico, some 150 miles south of Choctaw County. The practice was a busy one, and it dealt with all animal species, but I had spent the majority of my time working with cows.

I felt that I could make it on my own because of the training and experience from these practices, plus my farm background working with livestock.

My parents owned and operated a small general farm in middle Tennessee where we milked cows, raised hogs and chickens, and grew cotton, small grains, and hay. There was always plenty of work for a growing boy, from picking cotton to cleaning out henhouses to milking cows twice a day the old-fashioned way—by hand.

Even though there was a constant string of daily chores, my parents had insisted that schoolwork and extracurricular activities take a high priority. Sometimes it was difficult fitting it all into my schedule, but I was to find later that a tight schedule as a teenager was good training for a busy adult life.

My folks placed great value on a college degree and service to mankind. They had both spent a year or so in college, but in their era money was scarce and they were never able to obtain their degrees. My mother wanted me to study medicine and become an M.D. I wanted to be involved with agriculture in some way, perhaps not through farming but as some sort of agricultural advisor. As a teen, I envisioned becoming a county extension agent, a teacher of agriculture, a soil conservation specialist, or even an agricultural research scientist trying to create new varieties of disease-resistant corn or cotton.

My early life was heavily influenced by county agents and agriculture teachers, and I went off to college with the help of a scholarship arranged by these leaders. It was in my first week of college that I became acquainted with veterinary medicine. My roommate was a preveterinary student and his enthusiasm for the profession quickly rubbed off on me, prompting me to register for the necessary preveterinary courses. I realized it was just what I wanted to do for a career. Being able to study and practice medicine and surgery, but without the awesome responsibility of dealing with human lives, appealed to me. Veterinarians get to visit farms of all descriptions and deal with all kinds of people, so I knew I could fulfill my desire for agricultural contact and scientific study.

Jan and I had spent many hours writing letters, talking on the phone, and getting leads from pharmaceutical salesmen about towns and counties that needed practicing veterinarians. After several months of searching, we had decided to move to Butler, Alabama, county seat of Choctaw County. We chose Butler partly because there had never before been a licensed veterinarian in that county. The economy was good due to the recent construction of a huge paper mill and a Vanity Fair plant, which made ladies' undergarments. But the only person we knew in the entire county was Mr. Sexton, the county extension agent, who had encouraged and facilitated our move.

It seemed like a nice, up-and-coming county full of regular, friendly folks, deer dogs, foxhounds, coonhounds, lapdogs, cows, pleasure horses, and millions and millions of pine trees. The only question I had was whether these people would support a veterinarian as much as Mr. Sexton claimed they would. I wasn't looking to become wealthy by any stretch of the imagination, but I wanted a chance to practice the skills I'd spent several years acquiring, and in return to earn enough to provide for the needs of my family with maybe a little left over.

In addition to making a living, I wanted my family to become respected members of the community. I wanted to prove to the people of Choctaw County, as well as to myself, that what I was doing was important and that it would make a difference. I wanted to show them that proper veterinary treatment of their livestock would help make the animals more valuable when sale time came, or preserve lives so they could remain productive and help a farmer avoid bankruptcy.

I was a little nervous about my age. I knew that some older residents would have a difficult time believing that anyone twenty-eight years old could possess a lot of knowledge, especially anything of practical value. They were certain that a lifetime of observing "hollertail" cows, dogs having fits, and colicky mules certified them for making quick and undisputable diagnoses. They could be right suspicious of someone who was strong on book learning but short on dirt-road experience.

Traveling on northward, I learned the names of the communities where I would be working. Silas, Isney, Gilbertown, Toxey, Melvin, Womack Hill, Needham, and Bladon Springs would soon become familiar names. We would soon know their inhabitants, the names of their dogs, how many cows they had, and how they really felt about their animals.

Looking in the side-view mirror, I could see Jan's head moving and her hands gesturing enthusiastically. I knew she was pointing out animals and various landmarks to Tom and Lisa, both of whom were perched on the edge of the front seat, hanging on to the dash. No doubt they hardly blinked an eye for fear they might miss something new in this adventure. I was so glad they were like Jan—always happy and ready to explore unknown frontiers.

It was late afternoon when we drove down the hill just south of town, then crossed the creeklet inside the city limits. People we met would throw up their hands, not because they recognized the overloaded truck and apprehensive driver, but because they were neighborly and it was their habit to wave at most everybody. Even today when a farmer in an old pickup truck waves at me, it kind of massages my heart and soul.

The town square was typical of most Southern county seats. An old but well-kept two-story brick courthouse standing proudly among oaks and pecan trees dominated the scene. On the east lawn there was the obligatory statue of a young Confederate soldier with his rifle standing forever silent, but reminding North and South alike that the senseless tragedy of the 1860s should never be forgotten or repeated.

My first stop, even before finding our rented house, was at Mr. Sexton's basement office on the south side of the courthouse. We stopped in the street and I bounded out of the truck and down the steps to the extension office door. There was a large sheet of paper tacked to the door with my name typed prominently at the top.

Dr. John McCormack, our new veterinarian, will be arriving on Friday ready to help you with your animal health problems. Leave your message.

Underneath there was almost a half page of scribbling in different handwriting, some in ink, some in pencil, indicating sick dogs, dogs to spay, sick cows, cows to be blood-tested, horses needing worm medicine, and several other requests. There was even a message from the Chamber of Commerce.

"Thank goodness you're here, Dr. John," declared Mr. Sexton when I barged through the door. "Folks have been calling this office wanting you ever since your announcement came out in the paper yesterday."

"I can't believe it!" I exclaimed, as he handed me a handful of messages.

"Well, you said you wanted a job. Now, go to work."

We were on our way!

Chapter 2

THE AGED HOUSE that Mr. Sexton had rented for us was less than a half-mile down the road from the courthouse, but the pavement ended abruptly at the town-limit sign. I stopped the truck and quietly surveyed the unpaved roadway, free of any substantial packed base, gravel, or crushed stone. Thanks to the recent rains, it was now a hopeless quagmire of red goo punctuated by various-size holes and trenches full of yellow-tan aqueous material. I didn't know it at the time, but I was staring at a state-of-the-art, 1960s Deep South, prewinter secondary thoroughfare.

Certainly it was not the first such almost impassable road that I had ever encountered, but this one was different. This road belonged to me. My family and I were going to live here and travel back and forth over this road, mud and holes notwithstanding.

I peered into the rearview mirror to see if Jan had observed the mess ahead. Apparently she had, but she seemed ready to drive because her fingers were strumming impatiently on the steering wheel. She was anxious to get on with it, to see our new home and to personally inspect each room, closet, and cranny.

Most Southerners are worthless trying to drive in ice and snow, but we do right well in mud. It may be in our genes, or perhaps it's because we get so much practice. So, using my natural or acquired skills, I directed the truck into the muck, slipping and sliding through the one hundred or so yards of county-owned right-of-way. My front wheels attacked the mudholes and geysered a forty-five-degree wall of dingy water into the frostbitten buckgrass and kudzu growing in the ditches. Fighting the steering wheel was the easy and fun part of the ride. When the truck started sliding too much to one side, I simply twirled the steering wheel as far as possible in the opposite direction. Then just when I felt the overcompensation in the rear of the truck, I turned the wheel the other way. Soon I was skidding safely to a stop on a few pounds of gravel that had been sprinkled on the makeshift parking area in front of our new home.

As I got out, the roar of Jan's engine and the clatter of the underside of the chassis scraping on mud and rocks echoed from the other side of the truck until she slid into the remaining parking slot. Tom and Lisa were acting goofy, as if they'd been on a wild carnival ride. It was obvious that they had not thought far enough ahead to anticipate the next trip to town.

"You OK?" I asked Jan. "I wasn't sure we'd get through that muck."

"It wasn't so bad. I just followed your tracks," she said. "It'll be better going back out because the car won't be loaded and so low to the ground." Presently we were standing side by side, staring at our new home.

The house was a standard rectangular-shaped two-bedroom structure, with a carport and storage room on the right side. It was covered with siding shingles made of some strange synthetic material, which had been painted a nauseous green color.

"Why it's phenothiazine green!" joked Jan. Phenothiazine was the name of the compound we poured down the gullets of cows to rid them of stomach and intestinal worms.

The lot on which the house sat was slightly higher than the roadway and gradually sloped upward from front to back, which made the small front porch of the house some six to eight feet off the ground and accessible by a dozen concrete steps. It was nothing fancy by any means, but it was our first single-family dwelling and I thought it was just peachy, except for the color.

"Well, it's mighty small," declared Jan. "But I'm sure it will do just fine."

I would find out later that no building is ever big enough for the woman of the house. I think it has something to do with the nest-building instinct inherent in the female genes of the species.

"Daddy, the front door is open," announced Tom, as he disappeared inside, followed by a much slower Lisa, who was having a little difficulty maneuvering up the steps.

Tom appointed himself tour guide and presently he was pointing out all the positive features of the house, but saying nothing about the negatives.

"Momma and Daddy, this is your bedroom," he announced when we reached the end of the hall. "Lisa and I will take this one over here." Even at that early age I knew that his gift of gab would some-day serve him well. Perhaps he would become a lawyer or politician. "And here's the bathroom."

Now a more experienced Jan took over from the amateurish Tom. The way she went into action reminded me of a top general who was inspecting his newly acquired headquarters for the first time. Like jumpy flunkies in her wake, the children and I were in awe of her ability to detect so many interior decorating disfigurements that escaped our less-seasoned eyes. However, once she pointed out the obvious, I wondered how I could have missed them.

Somehow, I think men are less observant about the inside of a house than are women. While the women are inspecting the condition of the doorjambs and looking for mouse droppings, we men are trying to figure out where to set the gun case, which door to exit in a hurry to make an early morning emergency call, or where our wives plan to hide the iced tea glasses.

"There's a broken windowpane in our bedroom, the lavatory is leaking, and the showerhead is broken," she announced, never break-ing stride. "There's a hole in the floor in the hall closet and the roof leaks over there in the corner of the living room. There's no place for a washing machine and I just saw a huge roach in the sink. Other than that, everything's OK," she said with a big smile.

"Isn't this great? We're starting our own practice in a new town," she added, happily. "We're going to meet all sorts of new and interest-ing people and animals."

"Well, I just hope they'll call their new veterinarian," I replied.

I kept imagining making farm calls, attending to calf birthings, treat-ing colicky horses, vaccinating pigs, investigating herd outbreaks of serious bovine diseases, treating the pets of children, and spending long days and nights inspecting cattle at shows and sales. In my mind, none of my patients would ever die, since my skill would always prevail.

I knew Jan was thinking about creating a healthy, stable, and happy home environment for her family, and wondering exactly how she would fit her community activities into her busy schedule assisting her husband with his practice.

Tom was probably wondering who his new playmates would be and what sort of devilment he could get into out amongst the tall pine trees in the yard.

Since Lisa was only two years old, I'm not sure she was giving a lot of thought to the new surroundings, other than being sure she and her dolly had a place to play. As I was thinking about how fortunate I was to have such a great family and a great opportunity, I heard a noise at the side door onto the carport. Peering down the hallway, I could see the figure of an overalled man with a wadded-up blanket clutched to his chest.

"What in the world?" I mumbled. "Who could that be?" Now he was knocking on the window and I could see the sad face of a young child through the bottom pane on the right. Like a rabbit on springs, Tom jumped to the door and opened it wide.

"Boy, is yo' daddy home?" asked the man, gruffly.

"Yes sir, he's right here," replied Tom.

"May I help you?"

"You the vetnery?"

"Yes sir, I'm Dr. McCormack."

"My name's Moseley. That county agent feller said you might could look at this sick pup," he growled, peeling away several layers of old quilts. "I reckon he's been poisoned."

There at the bottom of the quilt nest was coiled a small, skinny beagle puppy, no more than four weeks old. I could see a brownish-red diarrhea that emitted the foul odor of decomposed blood. When I opened his mouth, I found his gums were the color of skim milk—so pale they appeared almost light blue.

Then I looked down at the child. The pretty little blue-eyed girl was only four or five years old but her sad, dirty face and ragged dress plainly informed me of her family situation. No doubt they were living hand-to-mouth, were uneducated yet proud people who would rather die than receive a welfare check or any other form of charity without working for it. This was not the first such situation I had encountered, but it was the first of many that I would see in Choctaw County.

The puppy was suffering from a classic case of hookworm infection. The climate of the South is ideal for the life cycle of this dangerous parasite, whose infective larvae are picked up by dogs as they sleep, eat, and wallow around in the soil of their playgrounds.

The infected pregnant female will pass the worms on to the little ones she is carrying, which magnifies the problem. The puppies have no immunity to these parasites; therefore when they are infected with a large load of these bloodsucking worms, they frequently are somewhere around death's door twenty-four hours later. It takes dramatic treatment, such as blood transfusions to replace the blood loss, to save them. In addition, they need medication that will rid them of the parasites without being detrimental to their own fragile health. Thus arises one of the problems of treating deathly sick puppies. Too often at the first sign of canine illness, the owner foists some ineffective or highly toxic home remedy upon or into the sick dogs. This may be done for a variety of reasons. Some people feel they are financially unable to spend the money required for professional attention. Others refuse to spend money on an animal because they feel it is a waste of time and energy to call for assistance. Some think it is beneath their dignity to admit that they can't cure the animal themselves. Somehow they think it makes them less of a man if they ask for help. It is very frustrating for a veterinarian to see a sick pet that could be successfully treated and returned to good health, but be unable to do so, for whatever the reason.

Mr. Moseley told me that he worked at the big paper mill east of town and also owned a herd of cattle. This was the third puppy in the past year that they had tried to raise, and all of them had died because of this ailment he thought was caused by poison.

"Come on in the kitchen and let's put him on the counter," I suggested, "and we'll see what we can do."

As he placed the dog and blanket on the kitchen counter, I realized that Mickey and Go Back were still out in the truck. In the excitement of the muddy road, the new residence, and the arrival of the sick puppy, I had completely forgotten about them.

"Honey, will you go let the dog and cat out of the truck? Then maybe you can help me here," I said.

I knew what the puppy needed, but I wasn't prepared to do it there. It needed blood, deworming, and good nursing care for several days, but I had no way of getting all that done.

"Mr. Moseley, this puppy has a very serious infection with hookworms. He needs to be dewormed and given a blood transfusion," I said.

"Well, I've already wormed him," he allowed.

"What did you use?"

"Gave 'im some tobacco and then I got some powders down at the feed store," he replied. "So I know it ain't worms. Must be poison."

Many people have heard from friends and family that tobacco and garlic are all they need to deworm their pets. And it is hard for them to understand that just because they bought some deworming powders at the feed or drug store, it doesn't mean that they will work. They've just heard about "worms," but they don't know there are round-worms, hookworms, whipworms, tapeworms, and many more. Usually, the home-remedy wormer and the cheap over-the-counter kind are not sufficient for a severe parasite load.

Mr. Moseley's assumption that the pup was free of worms and therefore had been poisoned was a common one. It was believed that in every neighborhood there was a professional dog poisoner on the loose, who went around spreading poison indiscriminately. It was never known what kind of poison it was: it was just "poison."

Another misconception in cases such as that of the Moseley pup was that some depraved neighbor had fed the dog some ground glass. I always wondered how these horrible people actually crushed up the glass so that it would be suitable for feeding. Was it beaten with a hammer, did they pass it through a sausage grinder, or can you buy it table-ready at a pervert store? In reality, I suspect that very few dogs were ever fed ground glass in Choctaw County.

I told Mr. Moseley as tactfully as I could that the puppy wasn't poisoned and he had not, to the best of my knowledge, been fed ground glass. I also suggested that he take the patient to another veterinarian who was better prepared to handle this emergency.

"I thought you was supposed to be a real vetnery," he growled. "'Ain't they nothin' you can do so I won't have to drive that thirty-five miles to Meridian?"

I had a dilemma here. I wasn't set up to treat this puppy, but I didn't like having to turn away my very first patient in Choctaw County. Then I saw Mickey, our dog, panting at the back door. Of course I could use her as a blood donor, and I had worm medicine and other drugs out in the truck.

"Well, I can try. You understand that we just arrived not ten min-utes before you drove up. All my medicine and equipment is still packed up out in the truck. But if you'll leave him here, my wife and I will see what we can do," I promised.

The little girl and Tom were standing side by side and at that moment I saw both of them smile at each other. I knew I had to do my best to save that puppy.

Shortly, I was rummaging energetically through the truck, pulling out my black veterinary bag and several large boxes of veterinary paraphernalia, which I carried into the small storage room off the carport. Then I retrieved a large syringe and needle, into which I drew a small quantity of anticoagulant solution.

"Tom, catch Mickey, please sir," I yelled. "She's gonna donate some blood for Peanut." I don't know why I named the pup "Peanut"; it just seemed to fit because of his size.

Mickey had served as a blood donor on previous occasions, so it was no big deal for her. She stood very still as I raised her head up straight, clipped the hair from around her left jugular vein area, and cleaned the skin with antiseptic soap. She didn't even flinch when I eased the eighteen-gauge needle into the jugular. Within a minute I had the blood that Peanut desperately needed. "Give her a Coke and some cookies, nurse, and be sure she drinks plenty of fluids in the next twenty-four hours," I said to Jan, echoing what the Red Cross nurse always says after I donate. "Yes, doctor," acknowledged Jan, grinning.

Then came the hard part. When puppies are in shock, they are weak and anemic, as was Peanut. Their veins are partially collapsed, which makes a venipuncture very difficult. It then becomes necessary to make an incision directly over the vein where you intend to introduce the needle.

With Jan holding the puppy on his back, I made the incision, eased the needle into his flimsy jugular, and started slowly injecting Mickey's blood. After several minutes, Jan started twitching her nose and blowing upward with her bottom lip.

"How much longer?" she inquired.

"Not long. You getting tired?"

"No, my nose itches," she replied.

"Lean over here and I'll rub it with my nose."

As we scratched noses, I heard another noise at the side door. When I looked up, there stood a whole bunch of snickering high school–aged boys and a grown man wearing a cowboy hat. I'm sure they thought the scene of two humans rubbing noses while injecting a large syringe full of blood into an upside-down dog was some sort of exercise in devil worship or the practice of veterinary lunacy.

"Oh, hello," one of us said, as both our faces turned crimson.

"Uh, I'm not sure I'm at the right place," said the cowboy-hatted one. "Is this the new veterinarian?"

"Yes sir, that's right."

"Well, I'm Mr. Rigney, the vo-ag teacher, and these are my FFA boys. Mr. Sexton thought maybe y'all might need some help unloading your furniture and stuff."

"What a blessing!" declared Jan. "I'll be right with you as soon as we finish with this transfusion."

"Transfusion?" queried one of the boys. Now they were all easing into the combination kitchen/canine-surgery room and gawking in awe at the procedure.

"I ain't never heard of a dog getting a blood transfusion," said one.

"My Unca Bubba had one when he was operated on for an ulcerated stomach," replied another.

"Is that dog blood or people blood?"

A constant barrage of questions followed, some highly amusing, others dead serious and well thought out. It was obvious that they were being grandly entertained.

"Let's put Peanut in the bathtub, so when he makes a mess it won't be so hard to clean up," Jan suggested. We dosed him with worm medicine, gave him some iron, and offered him some of Go Back's cat food and whole milk from our cooler. The blood had obviously perked him up dramatically because he began to lap the milk and wag his tail a little.

Within minutes the Future Farmers of America boys started to haul in furniture and boxes. Since we didn't have much, it didn't take very long to get it all in the house, the beds put up, and chairs and tables temporarily set up according to Jan's initial plan, which could be almost guaranteed to change within twenty-four hours.

By the time everything was in the house, it was dark and we were all sitting around the living room drinking iced tea and discussing the role of the new veterinarian in the county. It was unanimously agreed that it would be difficult for a veterinarian not to succeed in the county at the present time. I wanted to believe them, and I did have confidence in my ability, but there were so many unknowns ahead of us that I remained only cautiously optimistic.

While we were talking, I heard yet another noise at the carport door. This time it was Mr. Sexton, who came into the house bearing a large pot.

"Thought you folks might be hungry," he explained, "so the ladies down at the office fixed up a big batch of chicken stew."

A loud cheer went up from the fifteen or so hungry voices. Jan wasted no time in digging into the right box and finding bowls, coffee cups, and anything else that would hold stew for hungry boys. As we ate and laughed in good fellowship, there came a yapping and howling from the bathroom area. Tom and Lisa ran to check out the disturbance. Within seconds they were back, each holding half a puppy.

"Daddy, he's a lot better, but he sure made a mess in the bathroom!"

"It looks like your first case in Choctaw County has been a success," Mr. Sexton said. "Perhaps this is a good omen."

"Come by the office Monday morning," he said, walking out the door. "I think I've arranged a sale barn for you one day a week if you'd like to work there."

Later, as I tried to get to sleep in the same old bed, but a different room, I couldn't get the day's events out of my mind. People seemed very nice and thoughtful. There was a list of people wanting vet service, and the possibility of sale barn work one day a week. Even though my conservative nature kept raising doubts about the wisdom of this venture, the events of the day indicated otherwise.

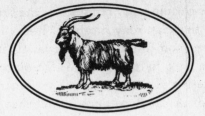

Chapter 3

THE FIRST WEEKEND in our new residence was spent getting everything in order inside the house. Mr. Moseley had arrived early Saturday morning to pick up Peanut, who had responded quickly to his blood transfusion and deworming. I knew that Mr. Moseley would probably go by the filling station and maybe the grocery store on the way home where he would spread the word about the new vet and the blood transfusion. I could just hear the reaction to that news.

"A blood transfusion to a dog?" they'd exclaim. "I've never heard of such!"

"What blood type is that dog?"

And, of course, the most important question of all would eventually be asked:

"How much did all that cost?"

I could just hear Mr. Moseley defending his decision to have the puppy treated and why he spent that much money on a puppy. No doubt he would cite his little girl as the reason, even if it had been his idea.

While Jan unpacked boxes and put away clothes, I worked in the carport. Since my intention was to spend most of my time practicing large animal medicine, I felt that renting or constructing a clinic building immediately would be unwise. It was also impossible since I had little money and an earlier visit to the loan officer at the Choctaw Bank had not been productive. Of course, he was very pleased about a veterinarian coming into the community, not only as a needed service but also as a new depositor. But since so little was known about the veterinary clinic business, no loan would be made for such a venture.

That's why I was cleaning and remodeling the storage room at the end of the carport that Saturday morning. It would serve as a tiny examination/surgery room until the time was right to move into a more appropriate facility. In the meantime, I would practice my way, and if my clients desired a more complete veterinary clinic, I would refer them to one of the modern ones in Meridian, some thirty-five miles away.

My little clinic had enough space for an examination table, sink, refrigerator, cabinets with working space on top, some shelves, and two cages. This setup would enable me to handle the routine out-patient cases, as well as keeping surgical cases overnight or longer if necessary.

I stocked the shelves with all of my familiar bottles containing the pharmaceuticals necessary for animal treatment. There was a variety of gelatin-covered, funny-smelling worm pills, each bottle containing a different color and size, depending upon the weight of the patient. There were injectable hormones, antihistamines, steroids, vitamins, and antibiotics. When I had finished arranging the counters and shelves I thought about how orderly everything looked, all neat and standing at attention in alphabetical order. I wondered how long that would last.

Tom and Lisa were constantly running back and forth from kitchen to miniclinic, trying to help. There were dozens of questions, especially from Tom, about what each medicine was used for and why. Then he wanted to know about each disease or condition that I mentioned. Lisa was also interested, but her attention span was short, and she had difficulty with the veterinary jargon.

Perhaps having children around the veterinary clinic or along on large animal calls is a little irregular, but it does give them an appreciation for the animal kingdom and the role animals play in adding to the quality of our lives. But I was to soon find out that having them near me at work was also great for me, since our time together at home was to be a great deal less than enough.

On Sunday morning we dressed out in our go-to-meeting finery and headed for the First Methodist Church of Butler. Some people claim they look better in three-piece suits, stiff buttoned-up shirts, and tight airway-obstructing ties. I am not one of those people. Deep down, I believe that everybody probably should go naked. That being impossible, the next best thing would be for everybody to wear over-alls or coveralls. They're a lot more comfortable and are much better for the respiratory system.

Nevertheless, Tom looked like a handsome little man in his blue suit and bow tie. Jan had Lisa frocked out in a frilly pink dress, com-plete with a pink purse and a couple of pink ribbons tied in her mass of red-tinged curly hair. We still couldn't figure out for sure what color her hair was going to be. It had that hint of red, but I was hoping that she would not be burdened with a lifetime of being called "Red" like her father. I'm sure that redheaded people will get extra credit when they finally check in up in Heaven, because they endure so much ridicule while here on earth. Jan was also looking right spiffy, in her one nice church and funeral dress. With so little money to spend on clothes for her family, it amazed me how clean and fresh she and the kids always looked.

The Methodist Church was located a couple of blocks south of the courthouse square, almost in sight of our house had it not been for the large woods in between. The red brick structure with its tall, white steeple reaching for the clouds could have been a church in Chat-tanooga or New England, except for the greater number of pickup trucks parked out front.

As we stepped into the vestibule we were warmly greeted, given programs, and ushered into the sanctuary. The center aisle seemed excruciatingly long, since we had to go way down near the front for an empty pew.

Going to a new church is always a little stressful for me. People are very nice to visitors but it's always embarrassing when the preacher singles them out and makes them stand, or sometimes he makes all the regulars stand but allows the visitors to remain seated so they will be less embarrassed.

This first Sunday was no exception: the preacher called upon the new veterinarian and his family to stand so the seventy-five or so worshipers could get a good look. I told myself at least it was good and free advertisement, since I knew that most all of those in atten-dance owned animals that surely needed some degree of veterinary care.

I could see Mr. Sexton about halfway back, probably in the same pew that he had filled for the past twenty-five years. I've noticed that churchgoers are particular about where they sit and I've even known some who make pew intruders get up and move out if they are sitting in the wrong place.

I thought the preacher, Brother Hastings, was a well-informed and forceful speaker. However, he appeared to be right provoked with folks who baled hay, hunted deer, and took care of routine weekday business on Sunday morning. And he seemed especially perturbed about golfers, fishermen, water-sport enthusiasts, and ballplayers who were enjoying their hobbies on Sunday morning instead of attending worship services.

While I was wondering how he would react to the practice of canine surgery or bovine obstetrics on the Lord's Day, I heard the distant jingle of a phone, apparently back in the church office. After the third ring a few people began to fidget and look around. Finally, one of the older gentlemen to our right rose and shuffled out the back door as the preacher continued his assault, now on cardplaying and cockfighting. About the time people quit staring at the departing phone answerer, he went into a tirade about citizens who spent their time over in those Mississippi state-line honky-tonks, drinking old nasty beer and smoking ready-roll cigarettes. A few people were really fidgeting now, some even getting flushed in the face and having large beads of sweat pop out on their foreheads.

Suddenly, the phone man popped back through the door and made a hasty beeline toward Mr. Sexton. A few words were whispered back and forth before Mr. Sexton stood up, looked around, zeroed in his gaze right at me, and started walking our way.

"Don't tell me somebody's called in here looking for the vet," I thought to myself, staring at Jan. She stared back, obviously thinking the same thing.

With a crook of his finger, Mr. Sexton summoned me to the aisle and then pointed toward the church entrance. Embarrassed, I followed, tiptoeing quietly, knowing every eye was slowly following the two departees. I knew that at least half the audience would have gladly shelled out cash money to have the opportunity to trade places with the exiting Mr. Sexton and the new vet.

The voice of Brother Hastings seemed to intensify as we neared the back of the church, probably trying to be certain the two sinners on their way out heard his attack on folks who watched professional football on Sunday. Once outside, we silently descended the concrete steps where we could converse in peace.

"John, Waldo and Kathy King have a problem with a cow trying to calve, and they need you as quickly as possible. I thought if you could go on down there now, I'll see that Jan and the kids get home," he allowed. "Now let me give you directions to the farm."

Good old Mr. Sexton. He had gone way beyond his duty as a public servant to help me and I did appreciate it, even though it was Sunday and I was attired in my best and only suit.

After he had written down the directions on the back of a blank check, he pointed south. "Better get going," he said.

I wanted to tell Jan where I was going, but I knew going back into the churchhouse would create another disturbance, and I feared that the riled-up preacher might single me out for a tongue-lashing. Reluctantly then, I left my family in Mr. Sexton's hands and pointed my car in the direction of the King farm.

"This is an odd way to start a large animal practice," I thought to myself, as I eased out of the gravel parking lot. "I wonder if being called out of church the first Sunday is some kind of an omen."

This was not the way my learned vet school professors said my first call was going to be. I had hoped my first professional call might be a prearranged appointment where I would present myself on the farm promptly and properly, all dressed up in clean white coveralls and spotless, germ-free rubber boots. After touring the farm and observing the livestock, I imagined that my clients and I would spend an hour reviewing the record-keeping system and discussing the long-range goals of the operation. Finally, I would make a few recommendations on the spot, then follow up later with a detailed, several-page letter. Instead, I was cutting out of church on a Sunday in the middle of the sermon.

Some five miles later, I turned into the Kings' gravel driveway and immediately encountered an old barn. The house side of the barn was a covered corral, and I noticed quickly that there was no cow contained therein. Further inspection of the corral revealed a collapsed section of the board fence, complete with traces of bovine tail hair and fresh belly skin left on some of the splintered boards. My patient had been corralled earlier but had escaped.

At this point, my common sense induced me to change from Sunday clothes into coveralls. It's always a temptation on Sunday calls to try to handle a large animal patient without changing into work clothes. But that temptation must be resisted, because fouling Sunday clothes with barnyard substances and then asking a spouse to clean them is a terrible mistake and does not promote marital harmony. It was clear this job was going to involve some cross-country travel incompatible with my good suit.

Presently, I heard a shout somewhere over the hill to the east, followed by the racing of a truck engine and multiple horn honkings. Other shouts followed in between honks and I could make out a few of the words being used. "Fool," "idiot," and several other somewhat less complimentary words were yelled in profusion.

"Uh huh," I thought to myself. "That cow has got all nervous and addled, and now she's trying to head for the back side of the back forty. I guess I better drive on over there and see if I can help."

When I arrived at the creek crossing, on the other side of the slope I could see the heifer loping, with head held high, up the hill alongside the east fence. I observed a small foot and head protruding from beneath her tail.

A high-headed cow in labor always means trouble and this one was no exception. When she reached the southeast corner of the fence she thought seriously about jumping over it, but for some reason changed her mind, turned around, and started loping back the way she had come.

By this time, all the yelling and horn honking had signaled to the neighbors that something unusual was going on in the King pasture. Men in shorts and a couple of women in aprons appeared out of nowhere. In minutes I counted twelve stick-toting Good Samaritans walking and jogging through the fields and woods.

"Hello, I'm the veterinarian!" I yelled at a man jogging by. He seemed to be in charge because he was yelling the loudest, barking out the most orders and calling the cow by the most uncomplimentary names. I assumed he was Waldo. "Can I help?"

"Yeah, come on with us," he puffed. "Bring your lariat with you."

Some thirty minutes and two passes by the barn later, we were no closer to having the cow corralled. The patient and her human pursuers were nearing the point of exhaustion, as evidenced by all the puffing, sweating, and side holding that was going on.

"She's headed for the lake!" shouted the one that I had identified as Waldo. "We'll trap her in the corner, then let the veterinary lasso 'er! You can throw that rope, can't you, feller?"

All twelve hands, two pickup trucks, four dogs, and one motorcycle with a busted muffler and a milk crate on the back immediately charged in that direction, kicking up great clouds of dust.

"Sure, let ole Doc rope 'er," I fussed to myself. "That is, if he can get within thirty feet of the idiot. Then if he misses, his name'll be mud! I'll just have to make it my best throw."

Sure enough, just as Waldo had predicted, the perturbed cow made tracks right into the spot where the lake made a thirty-degree angle with a new fence. She stopped, looked around at her pursuers, then quickly flopped down like an exhausted dog.

"Oh no, she's fixin' to die!" yelled a lady, as she clapped her hands over her mouth.

"No, no, Kathy, she's just had a labor pain and she's gonna give it one more try," said one of the Good Samaritan neighbors. He was a big, barrel-chested boy, and he looked like his name should have been Bubba.

"Go on! Git 'er! Rope 'er while she's down!" someone urged, motioning to me.

"Yeah, make haste, before she gets up!"

"Don't miss 'er, Doc," someone yelled helpfully as I eased forward. At least I had a good rope. It was one of those fancy nylon jobs like real cowboys have, except it had a quick-release device braided into its end.

Luckily, the cow was paying more attention to her immediate and distressing obstetrical condition than she was to the figure that was cautiously tiptoeing into her space. So when the perfect throw sent the loop circling around her neck from twenty feet away, it took her by surprise. It must have been at least three seconds before she realized that something was wrong, and then only because every last one of the men, women, children, and dogs present rushed to get ahold of the end of the rope farthest from the beast. The dogs expressed their canineness by barking right into the cow's face. The participants were all yelling either congratulatory phrases to the roper or derogatory expressions at the ropee.

She came up in a lunge, as if massive bedsprings had been glued to the bottoms of her hooves. When she returned to earth, her rear end was stomping around in the mud at the edge of the lake, as she tried her best to drag the rope holders into the water with her. It was kind of like a tug-of-war game at 4-H camp.

Fortunately, one of the group had the forethought to wrap the rope around a small sapling which tenuously secured our position. However, no progress could be made in dragging the cow out of the water.

"To heck with it," I fumed. "I've always wanted to deliver a calf while standing in deep water!" So in I waded, waist deep, until I arrived just behind the cow and in good position for an obstetrical exercise.

"Doc, if you go in any deeper, you're gonna need some scuba gear!" exclaimed Bubba.

In spite of the deep and chilly water, the cow was finally cooperating by standing like a statue. Occasionally she switched her tail, which slung water upside my head and onto the spectators.

Compared to the job of catching the cow, delivering the calf was simple. The fetus had a retained foreleg which required a couple of minutes of manipulation and then a steady pull. As I pulled, the cow suddenly jumped forward and the calf popped out on top of me just as I fell backwards in the water.

Quickly, Bubba waded in, grabbed the little calf, and dragged him out onto the bank. Kathy quickly began rubbing him with a burlap sack, which stimulated his breathing and seemed to make Kathy feel a lot better. It was soon apparent that the little fellow was in good shape, in spite of the wild excitement of the previous two hours.

"Drag him over there, right in front of the cow," Bubba ordered. "Let's see if she'll take 'im." It is vital that the new mother "accept" her newborn by vigorously licking him with her rasplike tongue. This licking stimulates the calf to breathe deeply and attempt to stand. But she made no effort to lick her calf; instead she looked in the opposite direction.

A couple of the neighbors cupped their hands to their mouths and made calf bleating noises, in hopes the momma's attention would be drawn to her offspring, who was now shaking his head.

"Turn her aloose," ordered Waldo. "I believe she'll take 'im. But first, everybody but Doc get way back so she'll think we're leavin'."

When released, I expected the heifer would ease up to her offspring, then sniff and accept her new baby, and everybody would live happily ever after. Why would I have thought that?

As quickly as the rope cleared her neck, she did an about-face, plunged into the water, and commenced swimming toward the middle of the lake. Kathy came unglued, screaming for someone to do something to prevent the cow's imminent death by drowning.

"She can't swim! She's gonna drown," the lady cried. "Do something, y'all! Somebody do something!"

She was jumping up and down, running back and forth at the lake's edge, while the gathering of neighbors milled around, kicking rocks and looking at one another. Waldo and Bubba rushed to the lake bank and physically restrained the frantic Kathy from diving into the muddy lake.

"Don't worry," I stated hesitantly. "She can swim! Actually, cows swim real good!" I knew that not from my professional training but from a movie I once saw where a whole bunch of cows were swimming across a wide, deep river in South America.

The cow proved me right, since by that time she had made her way out to the middle of the five-acre lake and was swimming with the grace of a water moccasin.

As the multitude watched, the cow finally reached the steep bank on the other side. It was obvious that she was weak because it took her several passes to gain enough momentum to get up the bank to high and dry ground.

When Kathy saw the cow was safe, she deposited the little calf on the tailgate of the pickup truck and headed for the house, where frozen colostrum was heated and prepared for the newborn.

Colostrum is the first milk produced by mothers for their young. In the bovine, it is necessary for the newborn to receive this colostrum as quickly after birth as possible. This first milk contains antibodies to the germs found on that farm, which were picked up by the cow during her pregnancy. If the new calf doesn't receive colostrum, its survival will be difficult.

Many cattle owners harvest colostrum from cows that have more than their newborn needs. If this colostrum is then frozen, it will be available in situations where a cow rejects her calf or if the calf is too weak to nurse by itself.

As I watched Kathy work with the new calf, I was impressed at her nursing ability. She had warmed the colostrum to approximately ninety-eight degrees, then poured two quarts of it into a nippled bottle. She carefully eased the nipple into the calf's mouth and stimulated the suck reflex by putting a finger into the calf's mouth. Soon he was drinking with enthusiasm.

I learned later that Kathy had been raised in town and had never dealt with livestock until after her marriage. But watching her work with the new calf, I could see that she had more empathy for her animals than the average cattleman. I looked forward to working with someone who would go to such great lengths to save the life of an animal.

Later on that day, the momma cow regained her senses and rejoined the herd. A bucket of cow feed enticed her to the barn lot where she was reintroduced to her new baby. Soon they were both very happy with each other and neither appeared any worse off as a result of their ordeal. Late that afternoon, Waldo came by my house with a check and a report that the calf was doing fine and had been named "Pond Bank."

"Doc, have you ever done any preachin'?" he asked, just before leaving.

"No, I reckon not. Why?"

"Well, the way you dunked that little calf, I thought sure you must have been a Baptist preacher somewhere in the past."

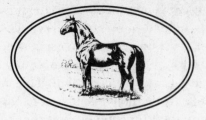

Chapter 4

THE FOLLOWING MONDAY morning, sunrise was greeted by the occasional blasts of deer hunters' rifles and shotguns somewhere out in the vast woods on the carport side of the house. Deer hunting in Choctaw County was mighty close to being a religion in the 1960s, and it continues to enjoy the same position of prominence even in the 1990s.

People hunt deer for several reasons. Some fill their freezers with roasts, stew meat, steaks, and ground venison because their families like the taste of it and it saves on supermarket beef. Others hunt only for trophy deer and are constantly having visions of bagging the Big One that has eluded the hunter's cannon for years.

Then there are those who hunt just because everybody else does and they love the festive atmosphere of hunting headquarters on organized hunt dates. They lug around expensive guns but have never fired them or zeroed them in like real hunters always do.

Some hunters are actually woods sitters. These people enjoy the solitude offered by the woods. They enjoy the sounds of rustling leaves and hearing the mighty commotion made by the feet of small birds as they scratch in amongst the fallen leaves for tidbits of seeds and bugs. They love the sounds of scurrying squirrels and jerky chipmunks, and listen intently to the faint sound of a diesel's groans as it advances its load of fine pine up a long grade a mile or more away.

The highlight of the sitter's hunt is when the deer come by. The pleasure is more in the watching in awesome appreciation than in the shooting. There are few things more enjoyable than observing the conduct of Virginia white-tails as they browse through the forest, their profiles almost indistinguishable from the surrounding trees and underbrush. Trying to hold completely still while a doe sniffs the air and stomps her foot at the unseen intruder somewhere nearby is a special moment in nature that too few people ever experience.

Perhaps a buck legal for the taking will come along, or maybe he won't. It doesn't matter; the nonviolent part of the hunt has already served the more important function of soothing the soul, if only for a little while.

About eight o'clock that morning, I drove out through our mud-hole driveway and into town, heading for Mr. Sexton's office. Already the deer hunters were passing through town on their way to work or back home. Occasionally, one stopped his truck at a service station where interested bystanders quickly converged and peered intently into the bed at the morning's kill.

I just loved the small-town atmosphere I was witnessing firsthand. Folks were waving and yelling greetings as well as insults to their neighbors who might be walking down the street or driving their pickup trucks around the courthouse square. They even greeted me, although somewhat more formally, as they tried to figure out the identity of the tall, redheaded stranger who was striding across the courthouse lawn.

Business was moderately brisk at the county agent's office. I've always had great respect for cooperative extension agents. The county agent is the local representative of the extension service, which was established early in the 1900s at all the land-grant universities. The purpose of the extension service is to provide leadership for agriculture, and to bring scientific advances to the farmers out in the county. The work the agents carry on, frequently behind the scenes, adds so much to the productivity and quality of life in the counties and communities they serve. There is no doubt in my mind that they deserve a large measure of credit for helping to develop an agricultural system in the United States that is the envy of the world.

As I entered the office today, the secretary was filling out the usual multiple government forms while a man holding a paper bag wrapped in string looked on and answered an occasional question. I assumed it was a soil sample going to the state laboratory for analysis.

A couple of people were at the publication rack, selecting and reading pamphlets on how to treat hog lice and the proper way to render out lard.

"Must be some new residents who moved up here from Mobile," I thought to myself. "Surely everybody in this county knows that a burlap sack soaked in burnt motor oil and wrapped around a hog lot sapling will do away with lice!" Well, maybe not, but just the sight and smell of it ought to scare off any louse that cared about its welfare and that of its thousands of potential offspring.

If you wanted to know how to render out lard, all you needed to do was ask the nearest neighbor. But first you had to get the hogs bred, fed, rounded up, killed, scalded, scraped, gutted, split, blocked out, and trimmed, and then pray for the weather to stay cold and the meat not to spoil.

The assistant agent, Mr. Deavours, was in his office with an over-alled farmer and his wife, discussing the merits of crop rotation. Like so much of the land in the South, their soil was probably suffering from chronic cottonitis. For years and years cotton had been planted in the same fields without any thought given to restoring the nutrients that had been drained away by the cotton plants. In addition, constant erosion of the topsoil had occurred to the point that the remaining soil was too infertile to grow much of anything except weeds and broom-grass.

Mr. Sexton was on the phone but waved me into his office when I appeared at his door. He was talking to someone about rosebushes and the need for timely pruning.

"Excuse me, Dr. McCormack, I have another call," he said, pushing buttons on the phone. "I'll be with you shortly." Then he shifted from rosebushes to Chamber of Commerce business as smoothly as a trucker shifts gears.

"Now then," Mr. Sexton sighed as he hung up the phone and rummaged through papers on his desk. "Let's see what I have here." The phones continued to ring and people continued to file by the door with various farm-commodity samples and reading material clenched in their hands.

"The regular veterinarian at the Livingston Stockyard is leaving for a two-year missionary experience in Cambodia and they need a replacement immediately. Are you interested?"

"Well, I reckon so. What do you know about it?" I replied. I knew that the sale barn would be a good place to meet ranchers and keep a finger on the pulse of the livestock industry, and would also give me an opportunity to make some money.

"They have a sale at one P.M. every Thursday. They sell mostly cattle, although there are always a few hogs that go back to farms and they must be vaccinated. There are health certificates to prepare, cows to blood-test for brucellosis and calves to be vaccinated and dehorned that order buyers will be sending to feedlots out West. It is a real good opportunity for you to meet cow people, because that's where most of the folks around here sell their cattle even though it's forty-five miles away.

"If you're interested, you need to call Mr. Billy Tinsley, who is the auctioneer as well as owner. He will probably want you to start this week," he continued. "Here's his phone number." He slid a sheet of paper over my way, with all sorts of information scribbled over it.

"OK, next item," he declared, shuffling papers until he found the correct handful. "Here's a list of county leaders that I think you should visit. Some of them you may have already visited or talked with by phone."

The list included Mr. W. J. Landry, timber and sawmill owner and breeder of purebred beef cattle and quarter horses, and Mr. Claude McDuffie, a respected commercial cattleman and valued civic leader. There were a couple of dozen other farmers and rural leaders, plus about the same number of prominent businessmen. At the bottom of the second page was "Mr. Carney Sam Jenkins, taxidermist."

"You need to make a special trip to see Carney Sam," he said quietly. "He's the best-known local homemade veterinarian and although some of his treatments are out of date, he is very popular and has a big following. He can be very helpful to you if you can work with him some way. If you alienate him, it will go against you."

I was going to have to give this meeting with Carney Sam some serious thought. Practicing veterinary medicine without a license and charging a fee for it was illegal, but I had to avoid any kind of confrontation with him at least until I found out what kind of service he was performing.

I knew from talking with veterinarians in other areas that getting into an immediate fracas with the homegrown animal doctors could be hazardous to the harmonious beginning of a new practice. After all, they helped their neighbors at all hours of the day and night, and many did it without charging very much.

"Let's see now, we've gotten you appointed rabies inspector, so you need to go by the Health Department and get to know those folks. The Cattlemen's Association is meeting at Garvis Allen's cafe next Monday night and we'd like for you to be there so you can be introduced." He handed me more papers.

"Here's the sign-up list of people who need you to do some veterinary work for them, and here's a county map." Still more papers were shoved my way.

"OK, now one more thing," Mr. Sexton continued. "You may know that I have a fifteen-minute noontime program on the radio every Monday. I would like for you to be my guest."

"Yes sir, I'd like to do that. When?" I asked.

"Today! Can you meet me at the radio station about eleven forty-five so we can do it live?"

"Sure, I'll be there," I replied. I was very surprised to see how much work this gentleman had done trying to help me get started. After all, he had only known me for about two months. He knew very little about me, except for what I had told him, although I was sure he had made a few phone inquiries.

"Mr. Sexton, I want to thank you for all you've done for us. You've gone beyond the call of duty," I declared.

"Aw, it wasn't much. I just want you here to handle all these veterinary problems. I'm tired of 'em calling here and expecting me to go out and treat sick animals. I'm a horticulture specialist, not a veterinary one. See, you are doing me a big favor!"

I left the office in fine spirits, because I believe having things to do is a great blessing. It surely must be boring to be idle and unbusy, at least for more than a few hours at a time.

When I returned home, I met the telephone man on the way out. I immediately called Billy Tinsley at the sale barn.

Billy Tinsley was what I call a "go-getter." This term refers to people who are fast movers and hard workers. They believe in finding work, getting it done, and then moving on to whatever is next on the agenda.

"Mr. Tinsley, this is Dr. McCormack in Butler. I'm the veterinarian

Mr. Sexton told you about. I wonder if—" But I was cut off in mid-sentence by his impatience.

"Yeah, yeah, be here at the sale barn Thursday, say about nine o'clock, and we'll get goin'. Got a pile of cows to blood-test. Bring some hog cholera vaccine, too. And your health certificate book. You know what to do, don'tcha?"

"Actually, this is the first time I've ever—"

"Well, just come on, we got plenty to do. I gotta go look at some cows." The phone went dead as he hung up.

"Well, I reckon I've got the sale barn job," I said to Jan while she sorted dirty clothes over by the back door.

"Oh good! How much does it pay?"

"Uh, he didn't say!"

"Didn't say? Didn't you ask?"

"No, he was in a hurry."

"Do you know where the sale barn is located?"

"No, he didn't say, but he wants me there Thursday."

"Well, how will you find it?"

"Aw, if I haven't seen it by the time I get to the stoplight on the square in Livingston, I'll turn right or left, depending upon which way the pickup trucks and cattle trucks are going."

Jan wasn't impressed with that answer, either. But she had long ago concluded that if we had been army people, I would have been infantry and she would have been planning and operations. She has always been more businesslike in our dealings with the animal-owning public, preferring appointments to walk-ins, and scheduling farm calls instead of "Well, I'll just whip by there on my next trip that way."

"Don't you have an appointment with Mr. Sexton and the radio station?" she suddenly exclaimed, while setting the correct time on a wall clock she was hanging.

"Yeah, it's nearly eleven forty-five, I'd better go!" After all, it must have been nearly a mile and a half up the road.

As I pointed the Chevy wagon townward, the mud hole seemed less threatening than before, even showing promise of drying up some around the edges. The sun was trying to beam through the cloudy haze that had obscured the tops of the pine trees for days. I was feeling good, encouraged by all the things Mr. Sexton had done and the direction he had offered. No doubt the sale barn job would contribute a substantial portion of our income, especially while the practice was developing.

In just minutes I was sitting beside Mr. Sexton, responding to his animal health questions, using my best grammar, and trying to pronounce all the words just right.

We talked about rabies and how I was the new rabies inspector, how I would be the new veterinarian at the Livingston Stockyard, and then he said that I was a specialist in treating sick cows. I was surprised when he went on about how he had heard that my other specialties encompassed boar hog surgery, treating mule colic, and working with hunting dogs. I was beginning to get comfortable when we received the "time's almost up" signal from the earphone-wearing guy in the control room.

Walking into the lobby, I heard the phone ring, then seconds later the control-room guy tapped on the window and motioned that the call was for me. I took the phone receiver from his hand.

"Is this here the new veterinary?" I heard a gruff voice ask.

"Yes sir, I'm the veterinarian."

"You know anything about sick stock?"

"Yes sir, a little."

"A little! That's all? Carney Sam Jenkins and all these other jackleg vets around here know a little! I thought a college-educated specialist would claim to know more than a little!"

"Well, if you could be a little more specific, maybe I could be of more than 'a little' help," I suggested.

"I've got this cow out at the barn that's been ailin' for a month or so. Carney Sam said she had the hollertail, so he split it and put salt and pepper on it, one of my neighbors bored her horns for the hollerhorn, and then I treated her for the tightback with a turpentine-soaked corncob. The wife heated some lard and I poured that down 'er just in case she'd been snake bit, and then I been givin' 'er some high-priced sick cow powders that I got from down at the co-op. What I want to know is, reckon there's anything else I could do fer 'er? I haven't missed anything, have I?"

One of the first things veterinarians must learn is diplomacy, because the above litany, or ones similar to it, were commonly heard in this profession some years ago. Fresh out of veterinary school, I was strongly tempted to criticize this caller, and his neighbors, for exhibiting a total lack of knowledge of animal disease. But I knew that those who believe in such things as hollertail, hollerhorn, and tightback are not going to reject those beliefs just because some animal doctor says so or can't find them described in his books. In some cases some of these folklore treatments even work, though in my experience they usually are not very helpful. But since old-fashioned disease diagnoses and treatments have been handed down from father to son, and from old neighbor to young neighbor, young veterinarians need to be very careful when going hard against this tradition.

The ailment that was thought to be the most likely cause of ill cows was called "hollowtail," pronounced "hollertail." In the first year or so of my practice, it was standard procedure to be called to a sick cow whose tail had already been "doctored." A devotee of the hollertail philosophy would diagnose and treat a hollertail case in the following manner.

First, he would examine the last foot or so of the cow's tail. Usually a soft spot would be detected just above the switch, maybe one to two inches in length, that would be devoid of bone or cartilage. He would declare that portion "hollow" and the cause of whatever ailment the cow had at the moment.

Next, he would take a hooknosed linoleum knife and make a vertical slit in the tail, right over the hollow spot. Then he would pour about two tablespoons of plain, uniodized table salt in a teacup, add the same quantity of black pepper, and stir well with the wiped-clean linoleum knife. The mixture was then packed into the incision, which was then wrapped with a clean rag. Some finished up the job by tying a nice big bowknot. Sort of a calling card, you might say.

Variations in the hollertail treatment were common. Some people used red pepper instead of black. Some poured the salt into the wound first, then followed that with the pepper. One thing was standard, however: the brand name. The salt had to be Morton's and the pepper had to be Watkin's. Those using other brands were risking their reputations, maybe even their physical well-being.

One of my problems in those early days was how to handle the believers in hollertail. Most of them had suspicions that modern veterinary science did not believe in this common malady. Whenever I was called to attend any kind of sick animal, the subject was likely to come up.

"Doc, you veterinaries don't believe in the hollertail, do you?" was the inevitable opening remark.

Answering this question was risky and required some thought and tact. If you said, "Yes, I do believe in hollertail," then they would be happy, but you would not be telling the truth, because your training and years of study had taught you otherwise. I always thought about the brilliant but stern and inflexible professors of veterinary medicine who had drilled into our minds the importance of an accurate professional diagnosis and treatment. Any reference to something as unscientific and unprofessional as "hollertail" would have been met with icy stares and the threat of a failing grade.

On the other hand, to tell a group of tight-lipped elderly men in Washington Dee Cee overalls that there was no such thing as hollertail was to guarantee being ridiculed back into the car and sent home. I just straddled the fence.

"Well, I haven't read about it in the book yet," I'd say. "But I'm only on page two hundred." That seemed to satisfy them.

Whether all this tail splitting, horn removing, turpentining, and drenching with weird concoctions actually has any favorable effect on the ill beast is open to debate. I have seen animals survive such insensitivities and go on to lead productive and apparently healthy lives. However, I suspect many others died because of all the needless manipulation.

"Sir, I suspect we are missing something on this animal," I said to the man on the telephone, "something that I can't put my finger on at this distance, but I'll be glad to drive out to your place and examine the cow, if you'll give me your name and directions to your farm."

After some hemming and hawing and negotiation of the fee, he agreed to the call. Further hemming and hawing indicated to me that he suffered from a common country ailment, a condition I call the "can't tells." In this condition, a person knows exactly where he lives but finds it difficult to tell a stranger how to get there. When he asked if I knew where the old Smith place was, I had to say I didn't. Then he mentioned where the old oak tree used to be before it was cut down. I confessed this didn't help me either. Finally, he gave up.

"Just come to Womack Hill, stop at the store, and ask the feller behind the counter where Buck lives," he said in exasperation.

A quick consultation with my county map revealed that Womack Hill was about fifteen to twenty miles from Butler on the Tombigbee River side of the county. So with great anticipation, I headed in that direction.

Womack Hill wasn't a city, nor was it even a town. You might call it a hamlet. There was a small country store, a chain saw repair shop, and a couple of abandoned buildings. It was obvious that at one time cotton had been the major crop produced in the area, since there was an old cotton gin next to the chain saw shop. But the gin was in a severe state of disrepair: its tin siding was peeling and falling off like dead tree bark.

The country store was the central point, following the pattern of every other small community in the area. There were a couple of gas pumps out front, a kerosene tank up on a porch, and a lean-to shed off to the side to keep the rain off the air compressor. On the front and sides of the building there were several tin signs advertising bread, baking powder, cold drinks, gasoline, even bowel stimulants and a proprietary product for female disturbances.

Inside, sacks of chicken mash and livestock feed and blocks of salt lined the walls. There was a large drink box, containing "co-colers" of all descriptions. In some areas, this is what soft drinks were called. For instance, there was an orange co-coler, a grape co-coler, or a root beer co-coler. Cold drinks that came in large twelve-ounce bottles were termed "belly-washers," so designated because of the tingling and churning that is experienced deep in one's innards after swallowing one of the enormous draughts.

"Wonder if you can give me directions to Buck's place," I asked of the storekeeper.

"Well, we've got several Bucks in the vicinity," he replied. "Which one?"

"I don't know his last name, but he's got a sick cow, and . . . "

"Aw, that would be Buck Tutt, probably Old Buck, not Young Buck. Young Buck just moved up above Butler. Are you that new vet I read about in the paper?"

"Yes sir, I'm the veterinarian. I'm supposed to look at Buck's cow."

"Yeah, she's right puny, pore thing. Can't get up, she's weak in the hind end. We've done everthing to try to cure what ails 'er," he related, shaking his head. "I hope you can help Buck with her, because he helps everybody around here with their problems."

"Is he retired, or does he just like helping people?" I asked.

"Well, both I guess. He served in the infantry in World War Two and got shot up real bad during the Normandy invasion. He's a real gruff-acting character but he's got a big heart, and just loves to help others. He even buys groceries for poor people with his disability pension money."

It wasn't long before I was easing down a steep, rutty road to Buck's log cabin, which I could see perched on the side of a small pine tree–covered hill. Just down from the cabin was a cleared pasture of some fifty or so acres, which ended abruptly at the banks of the Tombigbee River.

At this spot, the slow-moving river was about a hundred yards wide, and as I gazed at its natural beauty and the gray, frostbitten Bermuda grass pasture dotted with cattle of nearly every color and description, I thought this must be one of the most rustic, isolated, and beautiful places on earth.

I slowly eased up the short driveway to the cabin, listening to the crunch and crackle of river gravel under my tires, came to a stop, and got out. Then I heard the dogs.

There must have been eight or ten black-and-tan coonhounds out behind the house, tied to stakes with chains ten to twenty feet long. When they spotted the stranger coming around the house, at least half the dogs signaled my presence by barking, baying, and running in my direction, only to be hauled up and snatched around abruptly when they arrived at the ends of their chains. They weren't discouraged from their perceived duty, however, as they repeated the process again and again, each time exhibiting the same enthusiasm as before.

A few of the dogs sat quietly, moving their heads about, licking their lips, almost smiling, and calmly treading their front paws up and down as if they were in complete agreement with the baying and ranting of their associates.

"Attaboy, brother!" they were probably thinking. "Keep up the yappin'! I'm right behind y'all, all the way, even if I don't feel like carryin' on right now. Yeah! Hallelujah!"

I noticed a couple of the antisocial canines were still half asleep, but even they would open one eye occasionally just to see if it was going to be necessary for them to enter into the loud commotion.

A man I took to be Buck was behind the house, looking over into the engine of a 1959 Chevrolet Impala. There was no sign of the hood. I reckoned he had removed it for easier access or perhaps the driver just liked watching the engine work as he drove.

"Mr. Buck, I'm Dr. McCormack," I loudly stated, trying to be heard above the canine clamor.

"Hey, Doc, just call me Buck. I ain't a Mister." Then he turned toward the dogs and yelled.

"HEY!!HEY!!"

"Nice black-and-tans," I allowed. "You coon hunt much?"

"Well, a right smart, but not as much as I'd like to. You hunt? Let's go sometime." All I had done was admire his dogs and he was ready to take me hunting!

Then I noticed Buck's lame leg. He had obviously suffered a severe hip injury, probably in the war. It looked like one leg was a lot shorter than the other. "How can he walk the woods with a leg like that?" I wondered.

"I'm tryin' to get this car runnin' for the widow woman down the road," he declared. "She needs it to get to the doctor in Butler, even though she ought not be drivin' in her condition. Her heart's bad and she's got the high blood. If I can't get this thing to crank, she'll just have to ride in my old pickup," he said, pointing to a well-used old Dodge. It had dents in numerous places, which might have been the result of cow attacks or sliding into gateposts.

"Nice cabin," I said, as we walked toward the barn. "Sure looks well built."

"Built it myself. My brother-in-law insisted that I ought to have runnin' water and 'lectricity, so he came over and helped me with the wirin' and plumbin'. But I don't use that fancy stuff very much, except when I have company, which ain't often."

Minutes later I was bending over what must have been Choctaw County's skinniest bovine. Nearly every bone in her body was visible as she sat there, quietly observing the newly arrived figure who was poking, probing, palpating, and pinching various portions of her anatomy. Finally, I straightened up and shuffled around the patient, trying to come up with an inoffensive and tactful way of explaining my diagnosis.

"Well, Doc, is it the hollerhorn or the hollertail?" Buck asked from his seat atop an upside-down bucket.

Farmers frequently react negatively when the vet suggests that their livestock are improperly fed. Therefore, I have always tried to avoid making a diagnosis of starvation or even malnutrition in so many words.

Instead, I pick some synonymous euphemism.

"Actually, neither one," I replied. "She's suffering from a, uh, uh, chronic energy deficiency."

"A what?"

"The High Trough Disease, the Meager Manger Syndrome."

"What do you do for that?"

"You need to grind up some corn, add some cottonseed meal, minerals, and salt, then administer it to the inside of her stomach twice a day. Do you understand what I'm trying to say?" I said.

"Yeah, Doc, she's not only got the hollertail and hollerhorn, she's got the hollerbelly!"

"That's a pretty accurate diagnosis, Buck," I agreed.

"You know, Doc, I wanted to take up this line of work some years ago 'cause I like foolin' with stock. Tell me, would I have to go to any kind of school to be your assistant? Or could you just teach me?"

Over strong coffee in his rough-hewn kitchen, I assured Buck that I sure would like to have him work with me, but I was not financially able to hire an assistant.

"Well Doc, anytime you need help just let me know. Or if you're in this area come git me, day or night."

I thought about Buck as I drove home. I was amazed at his independence and ability to do things, such as build a house, repair cars, and give of himself to people who needed him. And he did all this, plus tended to a hundred cows, with a badly crippled leg, and asked for nothing in return.

"I think I'm gonna love these people!" I said to myself.

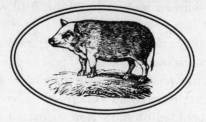

Chapter 5

THURSDAY FINALLY ARRIVED, and I was anxious to get started on my first day as the official veterinarian of the Livingston Stockyard some forty-five miles north of Butler. It was a cold day in Alabama as I drove up State Highway 17, and I reflected on the advice of an old family friend.

"Get yourself a sale barn or two to work, boy, and you'll have it made!" This sounded good to me since the veterinarian in my hometown worked two sale barns and appeared to be mighty prosperous. He was always buying farms, was chairman of the board at the bank, and traded every year for a new blue Ford. Besides, when I helped him work at the sale barn, he always produced a horse-choking-size wad of greenbacks and peeled me off one or two when the long day was over.

At the time, I didn't know that sale barn work was closely akin to professional football, in that both professions required one to "play with pain." I didn't notice that his knobby fingers were the result of them being mercilessly smashed between cow neck and head gate; or his hunched back caused by spending so much time bent over, jabbing cows in their right jugular veins; or the scars on his forehead from flying nose tongs prematurely released by amateur assistants.

By the time I arrived in Butler, I knew that sale barn work is dusty, dirty, stressful, and often degrading, but I also knew it would be an important source of income. At the barn my job would consist primarily of taking blood samples from cows to check for brucellosis, also called Bang's disease. The Livingston sale barn was an ideal center for checking cows since the weekly sale drew cattle from many herds throughout Alabama and east Mississippi. I knew that I would also be vaccinating pigs, writing health certificates, and inspecting livestock for shipment across state lines. I also knew that even though the working conditions were far from ideal, the pay was good and I would be around a lot of cow folks.

Having never been around a large group of cowboys before, I was somewhat intimidated by my first sight of the sale barn area. In the several-acre lot in front of the barn there were probably a hundred or more pickup trucks, trailers, and a couple of eighteen-wheelers, one of which was a double-decker. There was even a low-slung "possum belly" trailer, which had additional hauling space down between the front and rear tires.

As I drove through the parking lot, I noticed there seemed to be a truck pecking order. The bigger, newer rigs seemed to enjoy the closest, most prominent, and least muddy parking areas. The older, non-four-wheel-drive pickups with rickety sideboards or hitched to tiny homemade trailers were banished to the periphery of the property, some even parked on the side of the highway out front. Regardless of shape, condition, or status in the pecking order, all of the trucks had two things in common. They all hauled livestock of some description and they all emitted the unmistakable scent of cow manure, which quickly permeated my station wagon in spite of my closed windows. Some people find this smell objectionable, but it doesn't particularly bother me and I never go out of my way to avoid it. That has been a blessing, since at least half the work I do with large animals is concentrated in areas behind the last rib.

In spite of the cold, cowboys by the dozens were congregated out front in various-size groups, from two or three up to a dozen or so. They were nearly all attired in the proper costume, which consisted of huge wide-brimmed hats, cowboy boots, and old jeans that sagged down over the bootheels, so low that they were constantly being stomped on. Shirtwear was varied, and most were covered with a vest of some type. Many of the men were using tobacco, either of the chewing or dipping variety, and most were prolific spitters.

A few nonconformists, mostly from Choctaw County, wore seed company caps, overalls, and regular brogan shoes. The real cowboys were from the "black belt" of Alabama, a strip of black gumbo land that stretched from Montgomery west into eastern Mississippi. This area was better known for rolling pastureland and large cow herds than Choctaw County, where large tracts of timberland were more common.

As I drove my station wagon right up front near the office, all the cowboys and the Choctaw County crowd stared at my vehicle.

"The very idea," they seemed to be thinking, "this city feller coming up here in a car. And a station wagon at that! We ought to make him park way out yonder on the street."

I couldn't win! The cowboys made fun of my clean, family vehicle, but when Jan had gone to the grocery store in it on Saturday, she had come home with an imaginary clothespin on her nose and suggested that we ought to clean out the car for our Sunday trip to church. She was concerned that the kids might be laughed at because they smelled of hog minerals and bull bowel stimulants. What she didn't realize was that Tom and Lisa thought everybody had needles and dozens of cow pills in their vehicles, not to mention a cooler full of animal vaccines. They thought that a car was supposed to smell like a barn lot.

I sneaked out of the car, easing the door shut quietly and silently declaring that there would definitely be a pickup truck in my near future. Then I took my first real look at the sale barn.

The roof covered an area the size of a football field. Other than a portion of the front which was concrete-blocked for the office, there were no sides other than two-by-ten boards. It was one huge corral complete with cross fences and a roof. Ten-foot alleyways on either side ran the entire length of the barn, which gave access to holding pens on both sides. The auction ring was located just behind the office and when the sale commenced, cows were brought up the left alleyway, then returned to various buyer pens off the right alleyway. Loading and unloading ramps were located on the right and left corners of the front. I could hear the chaotic sounds of cows bellowing, hogs grunting, cowboys yelling, whips cracking, and gates slamming.

"Where's Mr. Tinsley?" I asked, and received more stares. Immediately, I knew I had committed an error in good-old-boy etiquette. Anyone whose first name is Billy doesn't want to be called "Mister." In fact, it is probably illegal to do so at a sale barn.

"You mean Billy? He's in the back sorting cattle," the head bookkeeper said, pointing. "You must be the new vet. Billy said for you to come on back where he is. He'll be the one doing all the hollering."

I fled out the side door and into the alleyway, which was occupied by a cowboy who would occasionally open a long gate and cut one or more cows into or out of the pen, using a rigid whip. Then my ears picked up the hollering.

"Wet! Wet! Dry! Wet! Dry! Whoap! Whoap! Watch that calf! Cut 'im off, cut 'im off!" an excited voice was yelling. At first I thought it was some sort of primitive preauction chanting ritual, the meaning of which was decipherable only by those persons who had passed through the mysterious world of West Alabama stockyardery.

As I drew closer, I realized that there was no mystery at all. Billy Tinsley was sorting a herd of cattle. The wet cows, those nursing calves, were being cut into one pen, while the dries, those who had no calves at their sides, were put into another pen. When the sorting was complete, the calves would be turned in with the wets so they could mother up. It is important for young unweaned calves to be with their mothers as much as possible at the sale barn, because of their greater susceptibility to infectious disease agents. The mother/child bond is especially strong in that species and involuntary separation is very stressful for both.

Anybody can buy a pair of irregular boots and a cheap hat and look like a cowboy, but you can tell real cow people by just watching them around cattle. It wouldn't be easy for a man or woman on the street to be suddenly thrust into the job of sorting wets and dries. However, a good cow person looks at udders and body condition; he or she has cow savvy and instinct. They know where to stand, how to move, when to move, and what to say. You can read the confidence in their eyes.

"Hey Doc, glad you're here," Billy said, as he kept moving. "Yonder's the vet pen, already got cows in there for you to test. You need to test everything on that side, pen twenty-eight on up. Got any help?" He was walking, talking, swinging gates, and manipulating a whip all at the same time.

"No, I'm by myself."

"OK, take Richard here, but you'll need to give him a ride home when you go. He lives on your way." Then he was off to another pen for more separating and culling.

Richard was a big, strapping good old boy who had dropped out of grammar school and gone to work cutting pulpwood, fooling with cows, raising hogs, and in general doing anything that would make a dollar. I knew at a glance that he was stout as a mule, but probably had little cow sense. I figured he'd probably get hurt.

Minutes later, Richard and I had retrieved our veterinary paraphernalia and were making our way to the vet pen in the back, where the wind was most vicious. The pen was loaded with thirty or forty waiting cows, most of which peered at us as if they knew exactly what was going on. The plan of attack was as follows.

Richard put several cows in the working chute. I caught the lead cow's head, took a blood sample, and put a permanent metal tag in her ear. I wrote down her number, age, breed, and any tattoos or brands on the proper government-authorized brucellosis test record. The cow was released, the next cow caught, and the process repeated until all eligible cows had been done.

The blood sampling went well for the first dozen or so cows, but then I dropped a two-by-four oak board on my right hand. I swathed the hand with soft horse leg bandages but it still hurt like blazes. Damaged worse than my hand, however, was my pride. Maybe good old boy Richard had more cow sense than I did. He was healthy and I was maimed.

After blood was drawn from twenty-five to thirty cows, the samples were taken up front to the "laboratory," which was nothing more than a vacant spot just outside the rest room. The blood was spun down in a centrifuge, the serum mixed with brucella antigen, and the results interpreted.

Out of the first hundred cows tested, thirty-one were Bang's reactors, and all were from the same ranch sellout. When the seller was so informed, he came charging down the alleyway to where we were testing more cows.

"What's all this here about my cows Bangin' out?" he shouted, "There ain't nothin' wrong with them cows!" He had a mouthful of snuff that sprayed out as he hollered.

"Yessir, they're positive on the plate test. Most of them are hot reactors. I'm preparing to brand them now," I submitted in my most professional manner. By law, all positive reactors had to be branded with a big "B" and sold for slaughter only, which meant a lot less money.

Upon hearing this news he absolutely exploded. Cursing, shouting, and spitting, he was preparing to take a swing at me when he inhaled too much dry snuff into his windpipe. Just as he drew his fist back past his crimson-colored face, his eyes suddenly rolled back in his head. He stumbled and fell, stiff-legged, up against the two-by-ten board fence and then onto the manure-covered ground. For the first time in my life, I had witnessed, firsthand, an acute attack of snuff overload!

Richard and I stared at each other, then at the carcass prostrate in the mud and manure at our feet. I was trying to decide whether CPR was indicated, and if it was a sin not to perform mouth-to-mouth resuscitation on someone with that much nasty snuff in his oral cavity.

I decided to temporarily pass on the mouth-to-mouth. After a couple of quick pumps on his chest, he began to jerk, shake his head, and spew well-used smokeless tobacco in all directions. His brother arrived just as we got him upright and together we half dragged and half carried him to the front office, in between spasms of gagging and coughing. By then, the guy was fully conscious and had a sheepish look on his face. He realized, I think, that we may have not only saved him from snuff poisoning but also saved him from sinking to death in sale barn manure. Nevertheless, he still wasn't convinced that his cows had any kind of disease.

"All this here fancy testin' is just a govmunt giveaway so you vets can git rich quicker!" he half whispered.

"Well, we gotta live too," I retorted.

After getting the snuff-overload victim stabilized in the front office, Richard and I took a short break to watch the cattle being auctioned off in the ring.

The ring was actually a semicircle surrounded by bleachers, with Billy, the auctioneer, sitting in a raised enclosure some six feet above ground level in what would have been the center of the circle. Around the periphery and in the first row or two were the big buyers, who bought for packinghouses or filled orders for feedlots in the states out West. But as the seats got higher the buyer pecking order descended. After the big buyers on the first row, the second and third rows would be commonly occupied by a few buyers and those cattlemen who had brought in a load or two of cattle, while the fourth row might be those who brought in one or two calves in their pickups. The last row was made up of spectators who were thinking of selling the next week, or some long-ago retired gentlemen from the old folks home who were engaging in the highlight of their week.

Observing the buyers making bids was interesting. When an animal would pop into the ring, Billy would immediately go into his auctioneer chanting and jargon. A few buyers, when placing bids, would simply raise their hands in classroom fashion. But I soon noticed that an experienced buyer would make the suggestion or a hint of a bid by the slight uplifting of a finger or a twitch of the corner of a mouth. When he wanted to bid no more, he simply looked up at the ceiling, yawned, or scraped manure off his boots as if bored completely out of his mind.

(Spectators had to be careful not to scratch or wave, because they might unwittingly buy something. When I reflect on the buyer and spectator pecking order, I recall the time Jan went with me to the sale. She sat on the top row, as dictated by sale ring protocol, but failed to observe the "don't move your hand" rule. Soon she was enthusiastically waving at our friends and clients seated around the ring.

"Miss Jan, you've already bought four bulls and I don't think Doc's got any place to put 'em," Billy declared, when Jan waved her hand for the fifth time. That ended her sale barn excursions.)

The remainder of that first day was uneventful, as sale barn days go. We got all the infected cows branded, vaccinated some hogs, and signed some permits and health certificates after just a couple more arguments. Richard talked me into stopping at the all-night truck stop for a greasy cheeseburger, which he swallowed whole and then washed down with warm milk. About fifteen miles down the road he suddenly developed severe nausea and threw up all over the interior of Jan's car.

"What in the world, Richard, why didn't you tell me you were sick?" I queried, perplexed.

"Didn't know I's sick," he replied through slobbering lips.

"Well, why didn't you at least roll the window down?" I asked, diplomatically.

"Thought it wuz open," he answered.

We stopped at a creek for several buckets of water and as we sloshed out the mess he had made I thought to myself, "Boy, are we gonna be in a car-cleaning frenzy this Saturday afternoon!"

The remainder of the trip home was made in complete silence, except for the whining of the tires and the lonesome wailing of the singer on the all-night country music radio station. Twice I snoozed off and left the road, once nearly decapitating a DEER CROSSING sign.

Arriving home exhausted, I looked in on two beautifully clean little ones sleeping peacefully, softly kissed their heads, and then crawled into a warm bed occupied by a half-awake spouse.

"How was your day at the sale barn?" she asked, sleepily.

"It was unbelievable," I mumbled, "and I can't wait till next week!"

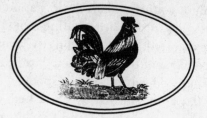

Chapter 6

I MUST HAVE slept in comatose fashion because I reentered the world of the quick in the same prone position that I had assumed six or seven hours before. The bracing aroma of Jan's morning coffee put my thought processes in motion, reminding me of where I was and that it was the morning after sale barn day, which meant it must have been Friday.

The voices of happy children and the tinkle of silverware encouraged my pajama-clad form to arise and walk toward the kitchen.

"What's wrong with your hand, Daddy?" Tom asked, staring at my bandaged right hand.

"What? Are you hurt? What happened?" Jan said, whirling from her position in front of the stove. She immediately commenced her inspection, checking both sides of the hand and then the exposed fingers for discoloration and swelling.

"Naw, it's all right, just banged it up a little. Just leave it alone. How about a cup of coffee?" I knew she would insist on medical assistance, but I didn't have time to go to the doctor or to a hospital for a passel of X rays and to watch them make a big fuss about a little broken bone.

"Oh sure, get an ambulance in here and call the fire department, too," I said. "Put him on a stretcher, stick one of those neck braces around his neck, and then..."

"John, you are just too cavalier about your health," Jan said sternly. "You take too many chances and you don't think about the consequences. Someday you are going to hurt yourself badly and then what will you do?"

"Well, I'll just stay here at the house drinking your fine coffee and playing all day with these fine children," I said, kneeling down and grabbing one in each arm. They yelled and giggled and squirmed as I tickled their ribs. "See, that didn't hurt my hand, so it may just be bruised!"

"John, you just don't care! I don't know why I bother!" Jan declared.

"Any phone calls yesterday?" I asked, as I spooned a double helping of grits onto a plate.

"Yes, there were. And I have made a couple of large animal appointments for you this morning. Let me get the daybook."

"Doing what?"

"OK, let's see. A man named Mr. Kent Farris called, and his neighbor, Mule Marsh, has a nine-hundred-pound boar hog he wants you to fix. I told him to get all the other neighbors to come over to help and you'd be there about nine this morning."

"What? Are you sure he said nine hundred pounds?"

"That's what he said."

"I've never even seen a nine-hundred-pound hog! Did you get directions?"

"Of course! It's right where the Melvin road turns off of Highway Ten. You'll see a big barn on your right and they'll be waiting for you there."

"Who else called?" I asked, loading the last of the grits onto one of Jan's big biscuits. It was oval-shaped on top, hence its name of "cat-head" biscuit.

"A young man who said his name was Stink Clark wants you to come by when you're that way. He just brought in a valuable bull from up North and he wants you to check him out. Thinks he has worms."

"Yeah, I saw that farm on the way to the sale barn yesterday. It's just south of Jenkins. I'll go by there after doing the hog. Anybody else call?"

"Had several information calls, asking the usual things. How much to spay a dog and deworm a horse, you know. Somebody called wanting to know how long a dog stays in heat, then a real nice lady needed to know what to feed orphan puppies. The usual stuff. Are you sure you don't need to go see the doctor about your hand?" she said again while staring at the hand.

"No, it's fine, and I'll go if I need to. Later!" I replied. "I got to go!"

"Daddy, can I go with you? Please?" Tom begged.

"No, Tom, there's no telling how long I'll be. Might be all day," I replied. "But I'll let you go with me very soon." I knew Lisa would also want to go, but at two she was still too young. It would be hard watching after two children while treating an unruly large animal.

Soon I was out in the makeshift clinic area in the carport, checking my black bag to see if I had all the necessary supplies to castrate a big boar. I needed my pentobarbital, which was the standard barbiturate anesthetic of the day, a surgery pack, an emasculator to clamp off the cord, disinfectant, penicillin, and tetanus antitoxin. I had the hog-catching snare, lariat, and the other ancillary items in the car.

In the South it was common practice for some backyard swine farmers to allow their male hogs to get to maturity before they were castrated. There are three reasons for the delay in surgery. First, if left sexually intact, a boar can be used for breeding the sows for several years. Second, he will grow to mammoth proportions, accumulating large amounts of body fat. After slaughter, this body fat will be rendered into lard, which is used for frying meats and potatoes at meal-time. In those days, the lard was just as valuable as the hams, side meat, shoulders, and sausage.

Third, there are those who look upon testicles from adult boars as a dietary delicacy. In the South, they are referred to as "mountain oysters." When sliced, battered, fried, and served hot on a platter, they delight the palates of some hearty individuals, in spite of their strong odor.

Restraining and performing surgery on a cantankerous barnyard beast four times my size is not an easy task. I knew from previous boar-cutting experience that this would be a big deal for the family that owned the patient and also for all the neighbors. It was likely that young boys would be kept out of school that day and some of the community adults would lay out of work claiming illness in order to see the big operation.

When I arrived at the front gate of the hog farm, I saw several old rattletrap cars, pickup trucks, and mule-drawn wagons pulled off the side of the driveway. The conveyances had no doubt brought specta-tors and self-proclaimed swine specialists. Some of the multitude were milling about, whittling, kicking clods, and inspecting farm equip-ment, while others were gathered in small groups, conversing animatedly. I was certain they were discussing the new vet, and what they intended to do if the hog expired under his knife.

I eased my station wagon carefully up the driveway, which was now dangerously narrow because of the vehicles parked on either side. I parked, then exited the car with a great show of confidence. I wanted the staring and now silent crowd to think that the white-coveralled figure who had just arrived in their midst was the foremost authority on boar hog surgery in all of Alabama.

"Good mornin'! How're y'all today?" A few nods and a few "awrights" were offered, but most just stared, almost as if hypnotized. I realized it was probably because of my white car, white coveralls, and my white face, all of which seemed highly conspicuous amongst the fifty or so black men and boys, not counting the women and small children who were occasionally sneaking peeks from the open front door of the shotgun house sitting back in the edge of the woods.

"Where's that big old boar hog this morning?" I asked.

Immediately every head turned, as if on cue, and looked toward a large weedy lot between the house and barn. Several fingers pointed in the same direction.

"Yonder he!" cried a young lad of about six or eight, as he too pointed the same way.

The lot was about five acres in size and was guarded by a fence of hog wire, old plywood, sawmill slabs, rusty RC Cola signs, and in some of the low places, small logs crammed under the fence to prevent the porcine inmates from rooting out. Thick dead weeds some three to five feet tall covered most of the lot, except for a feeding area near the barn and a half-dozen wallow holes scattered at random.

The centerpiece of the hog lot was a wrecked 1937 Chevrolet sedan up on concrete blocks, the inside of which contained old tires, buckets, and sacks. As I stood at the fence taking in the scene, a hen commenced cackling and emerged from under the raised hood, no doubt full of pride from completing her daily duty of producing a perfect egg. I surmised that she probably had a nest atop the carburetor.

"Whose hog am I here to see about?" I asked, looking around the crowd. Presently, a black man in overalls emerged from the group and eased over my way, holding his old felt hat in his massive left hand.

"Yes sir, I'm the one," the man replied. He spoke with a thick Southern accent, so that "Yes sir" came out as "Yassuh." I was immediately struck by his size. He was at least six foot four, weighed about 250 pounds, and had arms the size of stovepipes.

"I'm Dr. McCormack, the veterinarian," I said, sticking out my hand. After a moment's hesitation, he gently shook the offered hand, but not with much enthusiasm. It crossed my mind that it might have been the first white hand he had ever grasped.

"Yes sir, I'm Mule Marsh. The hawg's right down here," he allowed, as he too pointed toward a particularly thick stand of jimsonweed and briars. I knew the hog was down under there somewhere because I could see the tops of the weeds shaking.

"Well, we'll need to get him up here out of the weeds so we can get him hemmed up and caught. Have you got any corn?"

"Yes sir, I'll get a few ears from the crib. Leroy! Go git a few ears of corn from the crib." With the speed of a whippet, the young lad who had earlier pointed out the location of the patient dashed to the corncrib and back again in just seconds.

"Here the corn, Papa," he exclaimed in his squeaky voice.

"Sooeee! Sooeee pig!" Mule yelled, with hands cupped around his mouth. I noticed he had put his old sweaty hat back on his head.

After two or three recitals of the obviously well-practiced hog-calling routine, I detected the faint grunts of swine, then the sounds of rattling dry weeds and the clatter of cloven hooves on the rocky earth. The racket sounded as though an entire drove was rushing our way in response to the announcement of brunch.

A few seconds later, swine of every size, age, and description came bursting out of the weed growth toward Mule, Leroy, and the few ears of corn. There were red hogs, white ones, black-and-white ones, white ones covered with red mud, fat ones, wormy ones, very young ones, and very old ones. There must have been thirty or forty in all.

"Where's the big 'un?" I asked.

"He'll be here. Ain't no need for him to rush, 'cause he's the head man!" declared Mule. The spectators all agreed by smiling and nodding affirmatively as they crowded up against the fence.

Mule tossed an ear of corn over into a makeshift wooden trough and immediately every hog present pounced upon it as if it were the last one on earth. Grain, hair, and saliva were being ejected from the center of the melee like celebration confetti.

"Yonder he is!" It was Leroy speaking, this time reporting that the head hog had walked onto the scene. The little pigs with the highest IQs scattered first, all except one, who made the mistake of being directly in the path of the monster boar, and he was quickly nose-tossed some six feet into the air for his error.

I was gaping in awe, not because of the big 'un's half-ton size, his deep red, almost black color, or because of the way he lumbered right up to the fence and demanded more corn from Mule. I was wondering how in the world we were going to get him restrained enough to inject the anesthetic.

Rushing to the car, I quickly retrieved my lariat and tray that contained the essentials for the operation.

The most important, and most difficult, problem to consider in performing veterinary procedures on large animals is good restraint. When working with swine, there is the additional problem of eardrum-shattering noise once the patient is caught. Hogs have the unique ability to scream almost nonstop without pausing for air, except for a split second every half minute or so. Any attempt at voice communication is useless. Therefore, all instructions to assistants must be taken care of before the boar is caught.

"Awright Mule, here's what we're gonna do," I ordered. "Throw him a couple of ears of corn, then I'll get in there with him, slip the loop of this rope in his mouth, and catch him by the upper jaw. Then I'll throw the other end of the rope over to you so you can go around the strongest post you've got along this fence line." I could hear the expected response of the audience.

"That hawg'll kill that man when he goes in there with 'im!"

"I ain't foolin' with that hog!"

"How's he gonna catch that big bo'?"

"He better watch them tooth turshes. That hawg's liable to cut him bad!"

"I ain't never seen a bo' hog cutter wearin' white clothes before!"

All these comments were to the point, but none more so than the last one. I would soon find out that white clothes look mighty fine early in the morning or in a textbook picture, but where there are real soil, real animals, and real-world people, white coveralls last for only a few minutes before they take on the appearance of a major disaster. I thought about that as I climbed over the state-of-the-art hog lot fence and ripped off half the right rear pocket of the doomed white coveralls.

"You ready, Mule?"

"Yes sir, Mr. Doc."

"Throw him some corn then."

Holding the nylon loop in the ready position, I eased in amongst the swine as the corn scattered on the ground. When the boar took his first big chunk out of an ear, I lowered the rope, encircled the upper jaw, checked to be sure the loop was behind his wicked tusks, then yanked it tight. Almost in the same motion I threw the other end of the thirty-foot rope in the general direction of Mule and his associates.

A split second after the hog felt the tight loop on his nose, chaos commenced. The boar instantly launched into a screaming frenzy at a decibel level comparable to a departing jet, although at a somewhat higher pitch. He was jerking, pulling, and snatching, realizing that for the first time in his life he was dancing to someone else's music.

The other hogs were getting riled up as well, and they started a loud, open-mouthed grunting chant, apparently to protest the method of restraint being used on the head hog. Some of the sows were rushing up to him and mouthing around on his body, while others were biting at my ankles.

"Get away from HEEERE!" I yelled, stomping, slapping, and dancing in an effort to escape further lower-leg trauma.

Mule, Leroy, and at least ten of their wild-eyed colleagues were tugging mightily on the rope in an effort to just stay even in this swine-human tug-of-war game. I could see Mule's lips working in a frantic order-giving manner, but all persons present might as well have been stone deaf, because no sound could be heard above the porcine pandemonium. The rope had been on the animal at least half a minute and the screaming had been nonstop. A foolish thought fleetingly crossed my mind, about what a good clarinet player that boar could have been; then I continued my yelling and kicking dance.

Finally, Mule succeeded in getting the rope looped around a fence post and some of the assistants slacked up and began looking at the palms of their hands. A nylon rope has a very efficient way of taking the hide off a person's hand when it is slipping.

"PULL HIM TIGHT!" I yelled, motioning that I wanted the hog pulled up to the cedar post as tightly as possible. I knew they couldn't understand my request, but they did understand my sign language.

Soon the patient's head was tight against the post and I went into action. First, I double-looped a large rubber band around the base of his right ear, scissored off some of the bristles, and smeared alcohol on the top side. Luckily I could see a large vein swelling up in the correct anatomical position. I quickly drew my sodium pentobarbital into a large syringe, squirted out the air and a drop or two just like I'd seen on TV, and carefully approached the ear vein.

Many times a veterinarian's ability is judged quickly by his or her dexterity in making venipunctures and other technical skills. This was my first boar hog operation in Choctaw County and I sure did want to give the staring audience the impression that I was good at what I was there for.

The squealing reached a higher level when the new twenty-gauge, one-inch needle miraculously eased into the standing vein, and blood flowed back into my syringe as I kicked backward at the annoying pigs around my ankles. I carefully cut the rubber band and injected approximately three-fourths of the anesthetic, then removed the syringe from the needle, leaving the needle in the ear. After a few seconds, the squealing began to subside and the huge beast slowly went to his knees and then over on his left side. I was trying to hold on to the ear to preserve the needle in its proper location now that the boar was motionless. Occasionally, he took a deep breath, attempted to shake his head, and made tentative mouth movements. Blessed quiet had now descended upon the pigsty. I also noticed that nothing was trying to eat my ankles.

"Let the rope go!" I yelled. I slipped it off his nose and the chomping movements ceased.

"Leroy, bring me a bucket of water," I requested. Leroy sprinted to the well and soon had the water at the patient's side. I dumped in some blue disinfectant, then dropped in the instruments.

"He's a tough old dude, isn't he!" I said. It's always good practice to compliment people's animals, as long as you use the right adjectives. Cats are cute, dogs are splendid, horses are beautiful, but hogs are tough.

"Yes sir, he sure is," they all agreed, almost in choirlike unison. A lot of giggling and animated conversation ensued. Some were certain that he'd never wake up, while others were awestruck with the idea of using sleep medicine on an animal.

"Just like the folks' hospital!" I heard one man declare. "That hawg's dreamin' about bein' knee deep in slop." More laughter ensued, and even a few deep guffaws could be heard when they thought about the imaginary slop scene.

My examination of the patient revealed that he was in a very light stage of anesthesia. He still had an active eye wink and reacted quickly to a toe pinch. So I carefully reattached syringe to needle and injected the remainder of the dosage.

"Y'all can come on in here where you can see better if you'd like," I announced, while tying up the patient's top hind leg and exposing the surgical field.

I ripped a wad of cotton off a roll, dipped it in the blue solution, and thoroughly washed the scrotal area, then washed my hands. When I picked up the scalpel, a hush fell over the throng of thirty now arranged in a large circle around the surgical arena. On my knees and with blade poised in midair, I quickly scanned the frozen faces in the crowd, and wondered what their reaction was going to be as they witnessed the events of the next few minutes.

I grasped the base of the football-size right testicle in my left hand and forced it upward so the skin was taut and free of wrinkles. Then with a steady stroke of the scalpel I made a ten-inch-long incision over the top of the testicle. The incised tissue quivered slightly and the patient's tail slapped the ground vigorously before I managed to shift my position and secure it under my rubber boot. The involuntary skin movement and tail flopping told me that my anesthesia was just right, since the margin of safety is very narrow in a hog.

It's always surprising how thick the skin of large hogs can be. Even though I had made a bold cut, I had not incised all the way through the inch of tough skin. As I continued to deepen my incision, small vessels began to seep blood as the remainder of the skin gave way to planes of fascia. Finally, the blue-white color of the big testicle and its covering membrane became visible.

I knew that if someone in the audience was going to faint, it would probably take place at about that time in the operation. So I again scanned the faces in the circle above me, and again saw the same gaping stares of wonder. Nobody had keeled over, nor did I hear anybody making coughing or hacking noises deep in their throats. But I noticed that Mule had his eyes tightly closed.

"Mule, are you awright?" I asked.

"Uh, I jus' can't look at bleed, Mr. Doc. The sight of bleed makes me feel swimmy-headed," he declared softly, while keeping his eyes squinted shut.

Somewhere off to the left a couple of stifled giggles invaded the somber atmosphere of the barnyard.

"I heard that!" Mule exclaimed, turning his head but with eyes still closed. "Don't none o' y'all laugh at me or I'll bust you open!" Instant quiet ensued as I turned back to my patient and continued the job of breaking the testicle away from its fibrous scrotal attachments.

After much tugging and straining, the huge two-pound organ was finally freed of all its bodily connections, except for the main cord. I reached into the bucket and removed the emasculator, which is necessary to control bleeding when the final and complete amputation takes place. I set its semicircular cutting edge around the cord, then, using both hands, squeezed the handles together until I felt the stiffening of my forearm muscles and heard the crunch of the cord being severed.

At that moment of truth and at the point of no return, I observed a figure creeping up to my right side. As I lifted the heavy testicle away from the surgical field, a large, dented-up dishpan held by some unidentified volunteer was quickly thrust under the organ, and with a ceremonious "plop" I delivered the organ into the receptacle. Then the dishpan disappeared back out of sight. I removed the other testicle in identical fashion, and again the receptacle was in the appropriate place at the appropriate time.

"There you go," I said, dropping the other mountain oyster. "Enough there for everybody to get a taste."

The watchers grinned while eyeing the twin delicacies, and I noticed that a couple of them were actually licking their lips in anticipation of the grand feast ahead, while the bearer of the oysters strode briskly toward the back of the house.

The big hog, now several pounds lighter, continued his deep sleep as I inspected the incisions to be sure there were no tags of fascial tissue that would interfere with healing. Since castration wounds in large animals are not sutured, I thoroughly swabbed the area and sprayed the incision sites with fly spray. A quick injection of penicillin and a dose of tetanus antitoxin finished the job.

As I washed my hands in the blue water, Mule eased around behind the sleeping hog, carrying an old tin can in one hand and a stick with a rag wrapped around one end in the other. Then he proceeded to dip the miniature moplike device into the can and smear something gooey into and onto the surgical field.

"What are you mopping on there, Mule?"

"Just some lard to keep 'im from gettin' sore," he replied. He pronounced it "lahd."

"Lard will keep him from getting sore?"

"Yes sir, and it'll keep the flies off 'im too," he declared.

At that point, I felt sorry for the patient, not because of the surgery, but I was thinking about how horribly uncomfortable he was soon going to be, trying to walk around with all that greasy mess gumming up his crotch. Poor beast!

"Oh, yes sir, this here lard will help it a lot. It's good for any kind of swellin' or sprain," Mule declared. The hog lard treatment was another addition to the list of folk remedies that I was quickly learning about.

The crowd was beginning to disperse, but they were all talking animatedly about the big operation they had just observed. They were shaking their heads, gesturing wildly, and probably continuing to be amazed that hogs could be put to sleep just like people.

Mule and I settled up on the bill and I gave him aftercare instructions and suggestions.

"Now he's gonna sleep a couple of more hours," I told him. "And when he wakes up, he'll flop around some and be staggery for the rest of the day. Be sure you keep something on him to keep the flies off. Let me know if he swells up too big. You understand what I mean, Mule?"

"Yes sir, I understan'. He won't swell much 'cause I checked to be sure the sign of the moon was right. And I'll keep plenty of lard smeared on 'im for the flies."

As I drove down the driveway I peered into the rearview mirror. The remainder of the group was standing over the hog, examining the just-completed job. Mule was meticulously mopping on more lard.

I wondered why they hadn't taught me in veterinary school about operating in the right phase of the moon and the medical uses of hog lard. I guess that's why they said we'd be lifelong learners!

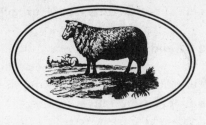

Chapter 7

BACK AT THE paved road, I turned right and headed in the opposite direction from which I had come. I was thinking about my next call, and the guy who went by the name of "Stink" and thought his bull had worms.

I had observed that lots of folks seemed to think that "worms" caused problems in their animals. It seemed to me that it was an overused diagnosis, especially when worms were blamed for everything from blackleg to broken legs to breech births.

As I accelerated the car and pondered diagnostic possibilities for the unseen bull, I observed a young man of high school age sprinting down the driveway of the farmhouse next door. Presently he was standing beside an aged locust post with a mailbox perched atop. I thought the curves in the gnarled post cantilevered the mailbox out dangerously close to the edge of the pavement.

The mailbox gave no clue as to the identity of the dwellers in the big house on the hill, but I assumed it was Mr. Kent Farris and his family. Jan said that Mr. Kent had made the phone call that brought me to Mule's place for the boar hog surgery.

As I neared the driveway, the overalled boy started waving his arm wildly, as though he were trying to flag down a bus to the city.

"You the cow doctor?" he said, stone-faced.

"Yes, I'm the veterinarian," I answered, trying to smile.

"Poppa said he wants you to look at a coupla cows that ain't doin' right," he drawled.

"Sure, be glad to," I exclaimed. "You want to ride back up to the house with me?"

"Naw, I'll just walk." Then he turned and sprinted back up the hill in speedy fashion.

As I drove the two hundred yards up the rough and rutted driveway, I observed the lithe young man and his seemingly effortless run. He was about six feet tall, weighed about two hundred pounds, and appeared to be all muscle. His overalls were a size or so too small, and the sleeves of his red flannel shirt were rolled up high, revealing his bulging biceps.

"He's got to be the star halfback on the football team," I mused, "and he'll go on to play for Bear Bryant at Alabama. Maybe I can talk him into going over to Auburn if I can make a good impression today."

The Farris house was an old clapboard structure, and from its style and state of dilapidation, I decided it had probably been constructed in the early 1900s. There was no evidence that a paintbrush had ever passed over its exterior, and except for the red rust growing on the tin roof, there was no hint of color other than drab gray.

The floor joists rested on stacked rocks some two to three feet off the ground, which made it possible to see all the way under the house and recognize objects in the yard on the other side. It also made a good place for dogs to sleep, chickens to flop around dusting themselves, and a convenient place to store junk. As I peered, I saw all the above, and more, under the structure.

By the time I had rumbled up to the side of the house, exited the car, and eased up toward the steps, the porch had filled up with men and boys.

"You the veteran?" inquired the one wearing the oldest and largest overalls.

"Yes sir, I'm Dr. McCormack," I replied, sticking out my hand.

"Kent Farris," he announced. I felt the hard calluses and the crackled skin of his palm. A hand like that had toiled hundreds of hours doing fieldwork, probably handling a team of mules and a plow, or perhaps using a hickory-handle hoe in the cotton field. This was a man who was used to hard work, the end result of which was usually an inadequate financial reward. But I was to find that owners of those hard hands usually did what they said they'd do, and if the veterinarian or any other service person was summoned, the bill would somehow be paid. If a farmer felt he had been overcharged, however, there would be no invitation to return.

There were three other stone-faced males on the steps with Mr. Kent, but no introductions were made. There was an older version of the squinting athlete, carrying considerably more flesh, mostly in the form of belly fat. To be more specific, if he had been a hog, he would have rendered out more lard than lean. The other citizen was a scrawny, wormy-looking specimen, in the same fifty- to sixty-year-old bracket as Mr. Kent. I didn't know whether he was a brother, a neighbor, or perhaps just someone who dropped in looking for a place to go deer hunting.

"Junior, you forgot to shut the gate down at the road. Run down yonder and shut it right quick," Mr. Kent ordered. Like a shot, Junior was gone, his rapidly digging feet sending particles of sand and dirt flying backward in his wake.

"Junior sure is fast!" I said. "I reckon he's on the high school football team?"

"Naw, he's still in grade school."

"Oh, I thought maybe he was at least sixteen years old," I replied. Actually, he looked closer to twenty.

"Yeah, he is, but that fool principal held him back a couple years on account of him stayin' home and helpin' out around here while I was gone. Uh, let's ease on out here to the barn. Got some cows that got ahold of some poison."

As we walked to the barn, each man reached into the hind pocket of his overalls and retrieved a pouch of chewing tobacco. For years, I had observed that the protocol in taking a chew was almost ceremonial, although totally lacking in formality amongst seasoned chewers. This foursome did not deviate from the standard technique.

First, the opening at the top of the pouch is pulled apart like a coin purse, while it is held in the palm of the other hand. Then the downward-pointed fingers of one hand are introduced into the moist tobacco leaves. The hand used is dependent upon which side of the mouth is going to receive the chew.

At this point, some chewers sort of stir the tobacco around inside the pouch, using a modified salad-tossing technique, but on a much smaller scale and using only fingertips.

Next, all four fingers and thumb are used to pick up a quantity of tobacco, the amount depending upon how bad the immediate craving is and how much elasticity there is in the cheek tissue. Chewers with years of experience possess cheeks that would make trumpet players green with envy.

The desired amount of tobacco is lifted to the pouch opening, shaken, and carefully placed inside the desired cheek. Experienced chewers can get nearly all of the desired amount into their mouths without losing leaves or stems. Those just starting out frequently put more on the ground than they do in their mouths.

Finally, they tidy up a bit, by removing some of the longer pieces left sticking out of their mouths. No one likes to see leaves and stems showing. All that should be seen is a lumpy jaw. The pouch is then closed, rolled, and replaced in the back pocket. Some chewers, especially older ones, store their pouches in the bib pocket of their overalls, because they don't like to sit on their tobacco.

The members of the present party were all seasoned users of smokeless tobacco, with the exception of Junior, who arrived back on the scene in time to bum a chew off his brother. Apparently he had been practicing only for a year or two, because he spilled a great deal and had a little trouble getting the chew situated comfortably in his jaw.

My nostrils had detected the hint of a strange smell when Mr. Kent and I shook hands, but I didn't give it much thought. I just assumed it was the old dog on the porch, or maybe hen leavings in the yard. But the faint odor persisted as we all trudged to the barn. In fact, the closer we got to the barn, the stronger the odor became.

Once inside the big hallway of the barn, I glanced up into the hayloft, and instead of seeing hay, I saw numerous cardboard Coca-Cola boxes. They were the kind that hold four-gallon jugs of Coke syrup.

"Boy, that's strange," I mused. "Wonder why he has all those boxes. And I wonder if they all have jugs in 'em?"

"The cows are right out back, Doc," stated Junior.

"Now we're making progress," I again mused. "At least I've got one of 'em calling me Doc!"

In the muddiest part of the barn lot were two brindle, white-faced beef cows. One was down, sprawled out in deathlike fashion, her head and neck flat on the ground. Her abdomen was swelled to gross proportions, yet she wasn't bloated with gas. It seemed that her stomachs were trying to assume the shape of a giant glob of sourdough. She was entirely too sick to survive!

"That's it!" I thought to myself. "That's the odor I've been smelling. It smells like something sour!"

The other cow was standing, although somewhat unsteadily, and she was bloated like a blimp. Her eyes were half closed and she had what appeared to be a half smirk on her lips. As we watched, the downer cow suddenly and silently emitted several gallons of watery diarrhea, which was loaded with grains of corn.

"Say you think she got in some poison?" I asked.

"Uh huh, maybe some mountain laurel or buckeye," declared the older son. "There's a heap of that stuff down yonder on the creek bank."

"Be quiet, Lamar," ordered Mr. Kent.

"Looks like she might have broken into the corncrib," I suggested. "Look at all these grains of corn in her excrement."

"In what?" asked the neighbor.

"In her manure," I said quietly.

"Oh, oh yeah."

"Uh, I just remembered somethin'," exclaimed Mr. Kent. "I had a barrel of corn soakin' out yonder for the hogs. I bet they got into that. Yep, that's got to be it."

"That could do it. They overloaded their rumens with corn, then it fermented in there, just like a whiskey still."

"Uh huh," someone said. When I looked up, they were all silently glancing at one another and shrugging their shoulders.

"Can you do anything to give 'em some relief?" Mr. Kent asked.

"Well, let's pass a stomach tube on the one that's standing and see if we can get some of this stuff to siphon out. I'll need a tub of water."

"Lamar, you and Junior go draw up a washtub of water from the well. Git that tub we put sausage in out in the smokehouse."

I sprinted to the car, found the mouth gag, jumbo stomach tube, pump, and a box of baking soda. My plan was to pry the cow's mouth open, pass the two-inch-diameter, six-foot-long tube down her esophagus, and then try to siphon out as much of the rumen fluid and corn as possible.

"Why don't you just git her to throw up, instead of puttin' all that equipment into 'er?" asked Wormy.

"That's because cows don't vomit," I replied. Instantly, I regretted saying it, because I remembered hearing of a roadside herd of cows vomiting somewhere down in Florida.

"If she'd just tho' up I know she'd feel a whole lot better," allowed Lamar. "'At's what I do when I git too much to eat."

"Be quiet, Lamar. The man said cows don't vomit and he knows what he's talkin' about. Now hold that cow's head still."

At that point, I had the feeling that something was about to go awry. I had made the bold statement about a cow's inability to regurgitate, with which some of my audience disagreed, and then Mr. Kent had made the mistake of saying that I knew what I was talking about. Nevertheless, I started the huge tube down the cow.

As the tube eased into her throat, the standing cow offered little resistance other than gagging a time or two. From my position directly in front of her mouth, I continued pushing on the tube. After it had entered the esophagus a few inches, she belched a powerful blast of odoriferous fumes that made my head turn and eyes squint shut. Then from her innards there emitted a deep rumbling noise much like the sound of way-off thunder.

Approximately two seconds later, and just as I turned back toward her head and opened my eyes, a massive explosion of hot, slimy, and stinking material blasted into my face, all over my glasses, white coveralls, even my shoes. I could feel the small particles of corn and masticated hay as they peppered my arms and face. In spite of the surprise, there was no need for anybody to tell me that the gallons of foul-smelling stuff engulfing almost every square inch of my front half had erupted from the very core of the bovine's viscera. But, as expected, someone did.

"Hot Toe Mighty!" yelled Lamar, jumping back even farther from the scene of the colossal upchuck. "What a mess!"

"Boy, she tho'ed up, didn't she, Poppa!" allowed Junior. "I thought the man said cows couldn't tho' up!"

"Shut up, Junior! Go draw more water so this man can get cleaned up." Junior flew, just as before. "Bring some croaker sacks from under the house too," Mr. Kent yelled.

My initial reaction was to attempt to get some of the odoriferous ingesta out of my right ear and from in front of my eyes. Several dog-like head shakes slung most of it out of my ears and some out of my hair. Mr. Kent and Wormy had opened their pocket knives and were trying to scrape great loads of it off my soggy coveralls. As they scraped and I sloshed my glasses around in the now-green water, I again heard the warning sounds of rumen thunder.

"Get back! She's gonna do it again!" I screamed. Then just as the cow's head went rigid, I jerked the tube out and a column of the vile material again erupted and projected some six feet forward. Luckily, this time no one was splattered, except for the downer cow. As the stuff covered her head like a blanket, she simply flinched her ears a few times and moaned softly. "Oh Lord," she seemed to be saying, "why me? How did I get myself into this mess?" That was the same phrase I found myself uttering at the moment.

The standing cow had miraculously deflated like a pricked balloon. As I tried to wash and the men continued to scrape on my pants, she took a few steps toward a nearby pile of hay and eagerly grabbed a mouthful.

"Well, I'll be dang! I believe that cow feels better," drawled Wormy. "But feller, you sho' are a funny sight!"

"Yeah, he stinks too!" Lamar exclaimed, as he stood against the fence some thirty feet away.

I sheepishly stood staring at the cow as Wormy and Mr. Kent continued to scrape. Their movements reminded me of the way the hair is scraped from the scalded carcass of a slaughtered hog.

The cow began to move around the lot now, probably in search of water. I decided a few swallows might be in order.

"Give her half a bucket of water, Junior," I suggested, when he returned from the well. She quickly responded to the sound of bucket noise, sucked up all the water, then stared our way asking for more.

"Look here, Doc, why don't we try the tube on this down one too?" Mr. Kent suggested.

"Well, she's pretty bad off, and it might kill her," I replied.

"She ain't no account this way. Why don't you go ahead and try it," he said.

After a few more minutes of trying to clean up, we placed the mouth gag and introduced the tube as before. She was more difficult than the other cow because she didn't have strength enough to even hold up her head.

Suddenly, about the time the tube passed the three-foot mark, the patient's eyes walled back in her head, she gasped, and her legs went rigid.

"What's happenin'?" asked Junior.

"She's dyin'. Let's just get away from 'er and let her pass in peace," said Mr. Kent. "They ain't no need in foolin' with her no more."

Minutes later we congregated at the well, where Junior had drawn several gallons from the twelve-foot-deep, hand-dug hole. I quickly cleaned up, then changed into a spare pair of coveralls, which made me feel much better. An aura of fermented corn still surrounded me, even though I had almost grown accustomed to it. I was sure that Jan, whose olfactory senses were highly sensitive, would detect the aroma before I entered our house.

Small talk ensued during the settlement of the bill. Mr. Kent paid off in dollar bills from a long, flat purse attached to a belt loop by a chain. I noticed that the bills had the same fermented-corn smell.

"Tell me this, veterinary. I thought you said that cows didn't vomit," questioned Wormy.

"Well, she actually didn't vomit," I stated, in my most professional manner. "Due to the complexities in the physiology of her four stomachs, she actually regurgitated due to reverse peristalsis."

There was immediate silence. Through their eyes I could see the wheels trying to engage to decipher the medical jargon that I had just laid on them.

"Now see there, Junior," declared Mr. Kent, "if you'd just go to school and study, you'd git learned up like this feller here and would understand all them big words. Doc, I've bought 'im books and bought 'im books, and he still won't learn." Then he stared hard at Junior, shaking his head.

"I don't know what all them big words mean, Poppa," declared Junior. "But I saw that cow tho' up all over that smart man. If that's what happens when you git lots of book-learnin', I reckon I'd just as soon stay dumb!"

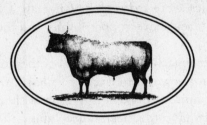

Chapter 8

I LEFT MR. KENT'S farm in a confused mental state. When we returned from the barn, there had been two newly arrived cars parked near mine, and two men were sitting quietly inside. As I wheeled out onto the paved road, a pickup truck wheeled in, almost clipping the suspended mailbox. The driver appeared goofy, almost drunk in the way he handled the steering wheel. When I looked back, all the men were going inside the house. What were they doing in there?

Then there were the other oddities. I was puzzled by the over-grown man of a kid who was still in grammar school because he had to stay home and work while his daddy was "away." "Away" to where?

Then I thought about Mule Marsh, the owner of the big boar hog on the previous call. It seemed to me that Mule epitomized the life and plight of the black man of that era. Even though the civil rights move-ment was in full swing throughout the Deep South, change would be slow in coming. Eventually, Mule would be able to sit on a bus any-where he chose, or use the same courthouse rest room as his white counterparts, and his children could attend an integrated public school. However, the economic reality for Mule was that he and others like him were hopelessly trapped in a world where they had few opportunities to improve their stations in life.

The paved road snaked through the rolling, pine tree–covered hills, pastures, and dry cottonstalked fields. Occasionally, I would see a "big house," then nearby, within walking distance, there would be one or more shacks, obviously occupied by black family sharecrop-pers. As I sped eastward, I wondered how many more Mule

Marsh—type families were existing in Choctaw County. I couldn't seem to shake the black sharecropper family and their life of poverty from my mind.

A few miles later I reached the outskirts of the small community of Jenkins, population a few dozen citizens or less, I figured. But I was impressed with the number of beautiful farms with improved pastures and nice barns. I saw fat cattle, sleek horses, and well-constructed pens full of fine hunting dogs of all kinds. I knew then that I would be spending a lot of time in the Jenkins area.

Jan's directions indicated that Stink Clark's farm was located approximately one mile south of Jenkins, and north of the Rudder Hill Hunting Club. I had already heard of the great deer and turkey hunting at Rudder Hill and the great pork barbecues sponsored by the club on special organized hunt days. It was a prestigious club, and membership was by invitation only.

I turned onto Highway 17, passed a prosperous-looking sawmill, and found the Clark farm about a quarter mile down the road. Pastures filled with cattle, a few horses, a red barn, then a nice brick home all gave the complex a prosperous appearance. Across the road from the house was a small country store. It seemed there was no shortage of country stores in Choctaw County.

I wheeled the station wagon into the driveway that led to the red barn, eased through the opened barn lot gate, and parked right up close to the corral fence where I saw a few head of cattle munching hay inside. Then I saw a young man of about eighteen loading bales of hay onto the back of a pickup.

"Hello! I'm looking for Mr. Stink Clark!" I yelled.

"Yes sir, I'm Stink. Are you the vet?" he replied. His voice sounded like he was about twelve years old, but his body looked more like that of Junior Farris. Stink was not as tall as Junior, but was a little heavier. He jumped off the truck and walked swiftly my way.

"I'm Dr. McCormack," I said. "Got an ailing bull, I hear."

"Yes sir. Daddy thinks he's got worms. He's right over here with these cows." He pointed toward a Black Angus bull about three years old standing in the corner of the lot. His head was hanging down and he was bowed up as if he were in severe pain. He was not eating like the other cattle, nor was he chewing his cud.

"Let's put him in the alleyway here and make an examination," I suggested.

Stink slapped the bull on the rump and he moved reluctantly, occasionally emitting an audible grunt. It was obvious that he was very sick, and it had nothing to do with worms.

Once he was in the chute, I took his temperature. There were no stomach movements and he was slightly dehydrated.

"Temperature is a hundred and four degrees. That's high!" I exclaimed.

"What's it supposed to be?" asked Stink.

"One oh one point five to one oh two point five," I said, "depending on how hot the day is."

"Do you reckon it's worms?"

"No, I don't believe so. He's too sick. I think he may have swallowed a piece of wire."

"Wire? Why? Where would he get wire?" Stink said.

"Take that hoe handle over there and stick it through the board here and then punch up underneath his stomach. Then I'll listen with my stethoscope and see what I hear."

When he punched the bull's belly, I heard a severe grunt right over his windpipe.

"Again," I said.

Another punch, and another grunt from the patient. That was enough for me to confirm a diagnosis of hardware disease.

Bovines are careless grazers and are prone to swallow nails and other pieces of metal, such as baling wire, because of their unusual method of grazing. A bull extends his tongue, gathers a wad of grass with it, rips off the entire mass with the assistance of his lower incisors, chews it a few times, and swallows. Later on, when resting, he will bring cuds of the grass back up and rechew them.

A bovine can swallow pieces of metal up to six to eight inches long, and these foreign objects come to rest in the second stomach, which is a honeycombed structure called the reticulum.

If the wire would just stay put inside the reticulum, there would be no problem. However, due to the movements of the stomachs, a piece of wire or a nail frequently pierces through the wall of the reticulum and into the surrounding peritoneum, which is the lining of the abdominal cavity. Because of the metal object causing the problem, the condition is commonly called "hardware disease." The official medical term is traumatic reticuloperitonitis, but it is a whole lot easier to understand if you call it "hardware."

I explained all this to Stink and then told him that we could surgically remove the metal.

"Reckon your daddy would want us to operate?" I asked.

"Well, these are my cows and I just bought the bull over in Montgomery at the bull sale. So I think we'll just operate," he declared, "if you think it'll work."

"How old are you, Stink?"

"Fourteen."

"Why aren't you in school today?"

"Had to stay home to be here to help you, didn't I?"

"Oh yeah!" I was surprised at how mature the young people in the area were. "Come on, let's go to the car and get our operating gear."

Shortly, we were standing behind the station wagon, retrieving stuff from the tailgate area, when I noticed Stink sniffing the air.

"Doc, I think I've changed my mind about operating on my bull," he declared firmly.

"Why?" I asked, stopping with medicine in both hands.

"Well, I don't want somebody who has been drinking whiskey to work on my animals."

"Who, me? I haven't been drinking!"

"Oh yeah? Then why do I smell whiskey all over you and all in your car?" he declared. "Isn't that whiskey I smell?"

"No, it's soured corn. I just doctored on two cows for Mr. Farris down the road and that's where that smell came from."

"Mr. Kent Farris?"

"Yeah."

"Doc, didn't you know? I heard he has a whiskey still back behind his barn. The ABC boys caught him makin' it and he's been out of the county for a while. His boys Junior and Lamar have been running the farm while he's been away."

Now I understood why Mr. Kent told me that Junior had not progressed well in school because he stayed home and worked. I also understood that the "soaked corn" was actually soured mash from the still and the cows had probably gotten into it accidentally. And all those people coming to the house were there to buy some of that homemade liquor. And I now knew why all those empty gallon jugs were in the barn.

I also understood why, contrary to local custom, I was not invited into the kitchen for refreshments after the bovine patients had been treated. Outsiders would not be invited into the house until they had done something special or were liked and respected enough to become an insider. Certainly Mr. Kent was not going to confide in me that he was a barnyard distiller and ask me into his kitchen to show off his full jugs of illegal spirits along with all those customers he had there.

With Stink persuaded that I was not liquored up, we went into action. I scrubbed and shaved the left side of the bull's abdomen while he brought buckets of water and two bales of hay, onto which I placed a large drape and my instruments. After the shaving and scrubbing, I injected local anesthetic into my proposed eight-inch incision line. I had to work through the two-by-six boards, which was somewhat awkward, but it was a lot better than having the bull haltered to one of the pine trees out in the lot.

Because most bovine surgery is performed on the standing animal under local anesthesia, the patient's behavior is frequently less than ideal, especially while the anesthetic is being injected. However, my present patient was so ill that he offered only token resistance. He stomped his left rear foot a couple of times as if giving some kind of bull alert, then demolished a rotten two-by-six board, which resulted in his leg getting hung up and wedged in between a locust post and one of the remaining healthy boards. I was pleased that he had used restraint when objecting to my chuteside manner.

It took us only a few minutes to extract his foot from its uncomfortable position and get on with a second scrubbing of the surgical site. Then I scrubbed up and put on sterile shoulder-length gloves. No more kicking followed, probably because he had worn himself out on the first blast.

"You ready, Stink? You've got to hand me stuff, but be sure you don't touch those instruments 'cause they're sterile," I declared.

"Yes sir, I understand," he exclaimed.

As my scalpel sliced cleanly through the muscles, the thought occurred to me that this was my first bovine surgical case in Choctaw

County. I tried hard to dismiss those amateurish thoughts from my brain, but they persisted.

"What if I get down in this rascal's viscera and there's no wire or nail?" I asked myself. "Or what if I get in here and there's all sorts of abscesses and infection?"

"Is he supposed to bleed like that?" Stink asked.

"Huh? Oh, it's OK. But I'll clamp that one off just to be sure." I was glad he had said something. It put my mind back on business.

One more nick with the blade and I was through the peritoneum and peering at the rumen, the large digestion vat that has the unique ability to receive grass, hay, and various commodity byproducts, then convert them into energy and protein. It is a remarkable organ, but it can't do anything with a piece of metal.

I quickly inserted the rumen board, a twelve-by-eighteen-inch flat plastic device with a hole bored in its center large enough to accommodate the right shoulder of a veterinarian. I brought the rumen wall through the hole, opened it, then everted and secured it with hooks to stainless steel rods driven into the plastic. This prevents rumen contents from contaminating the peritoneum and other tissues. Any spillage is directed to the exterior of the animal.

After the rumen board was in place, I carefully burrowed my hand through the rumen interior, downward and forward, toward the reticulum where I was sure the troublesome wire awaited. Everything had gone well so far and my confidence was building as the surgery progressed.

Large-animal veterinarians need long arms because they spend a lot of time trying to reach structures and organs that are located deep inside their patients. Even with long arms, sometimes the searched-for object is just out of reach, or can be barely touched with the fingertips.

This time I felt a long piece of wire lying on the left wall of the reticulum. It felt imbedded, probably sticking through the organ and into the body wall.

I carefully extracted the wire, brought my smelly hand to the outside and opened it up for the ceremonial presentation of the offending hardware to the owner.

"There's the cause of all his problems!" I declared professionally. "What do you think about that?" I figured the fourteen-year-old boy would stare at the hardware in openmouthed wonder, exclaiming something like "Gollleee!" or some other youthful phrase. Instead, he looked at it as if he were a seasoned cattleman, pondering the effect the problem was going to have on his herd.

"I'll declare," he said slowly. "I wonder if any of these other cows have anything like this wrong with them. Several cows don't look too good, and Daddy just thought they had worms. How long will it be before he'll be ready to breed cows? I've got to get a calf crop on the ground." I was not expecting such a mature response.

"If he lives, he'll be raring to go in a couple of weeks," I declared.

"If he lives! Hey, we've got to save this bull, 'cause I've got too much money in him. Besides, this is my FFA project!"

There are two groups of people who are dear to my heart. First, I love people who have gumption and try to accomplish something in life. Second, I am a strong believer in the Future Farmers of America organization. It motivates, trains, and assists young men and women in farm-related projects, helping them to develop into tomorrow's agricultural leaders. My appreciation of their philosophy may be due to my personal involvement in the FFA when I was a high school student.

As Stink picked through the smelly contents in my hand, staring at the long wire and fingering several other small slivers of metal, I realized that the survival of this patient was as critical to the two men standing there as it was to the bull. Stink needed the services of the prize specimen to upgrade his herd and make it more valuable. And since this was probably the area's first surgical removal of a large wire from a bull's stomach, a successful outcome would convince others that the new vet might know something about doctoring cows.

A second long-armed examination of the reticulum, this time with a palmed magnet, attracted a small nail, a couple of bent staples, and a gathering of harmless filings. At least the patient now had a stomach free of foreign objects.

After a quick cleanup, I closed the rumen with catgut sutures, swabbed it clean, then placed antibiotics into the abdominal cavity. I closed the muscles and skin and gave the bull an elephant-sized injection of penicillin.

"Doc, he don't look a whole lot better," Stink allowed as the bull trudged out of the chute. "You don't reckon he's gon' die, do you?"

"Stink, he'll probably get worse before he gets better. Just think about how sick he was before we cut a ten-inch hole in his side. Now I'll be by here tomorrow to check on him and give him another injection."

"What should I feed him?"

"You can try him on some grain and hay, but I don't think he'll eat much for a day or two. He'll be too sore for eating, walking, or breeding."

As we stared at the bull, a nicely dressed lady appeared at the barn lot fence.

"Are you the doctor?" she yelled.

"Yes ma'am."

"Mr. Sexton has been trying to track you down for the last couple of hours. He said you're needed to go up to Ezekiel Jones's place."

"All right. Did he say what was wrong? Do you know where he lives?"

"Something about his milk cow being down. Stink can tell you how to get there."

"Thanks for taking the message. I'll head on up there in just a little bit."

"I'm Dardanelle, Stink's momma. We're sure glad to have you in this county 'cause we've needed a good vet here for a long time. You're gonna have plenty of work, probably more than you'll want. I'm gonna leave you a piece of cake here on the hood of your car."

I didn't know it then, but there would be many more calls to the Clark farm, to work with their dogs, horses, and cattle, but none would be remembered as well as the "worm call" that turned out to be a "wire call."

"Daddy's gon' really be shocked when he sees this," Stink said when I handed him the statement. "Carney Sam Jenkins told him all that bull needed was a dollar's worth of worm medicine and his tail split with a linoleum knife."

"Yeah, scalpel surgery is a lot more expensive than linoleum knife surgery and worm drenches," I surmised.

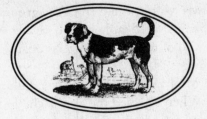

Chapter 9

EATING CAKE AND driving a car at the same time is tricky, but I enjoy the challenge, especially when the cake is as good as Mrs. Clark's was on that day. So with sticky hands and crumbs dribbling down on my coveralls, I headed northward to the Ezekiel Jones farm, according to Stink's directions.

Approximately six miles later I saw the big oak tree on the right where I was supposed to turn off the main road. On the side of the mailbox nearby, "Ezekiel and Ophelia" had been crudely painted. It was pleasant to see names on a mailbox for a change.

The drive up to their old house was difficult. It was actually an old dry creek bed, full of large rocks and holes, and it was better suited to being traveled by a mule-drawn wagon. Jan's station wagon was too low to the ground, and the undercarriage bumped against the rocks in spite of my careful driving. I wished again for that pickup truck.

Finally, some quarter of a mile from the mailbox and up a slight, tree-scattered hill, the house appeared. It was a shotgun house—a common Southern expression meaning that a shotgun blast through the front door would pass through every door and room in the house and out the back door without messing up a single wall.

In front of the house, I could see an elderly black woman with a blue bandana around her head sweeping the bare-earthed yard with a homemade broom made of sage grass tied onto a four-foot hickory stick.

A typical yard of the poor black family in the Deep South was characterized by an absence of mowable grass, but by the presence of several chinaberry trees and beautiful flowers. It was not uncommon to see the trunks of trees whitewashed from the ground up some four to six feet. Miss Ophelia's yard adhered to the customary standard, although it was devoid of blooming flowers because of the November weather.

In the backyard, Mr. Ezekiel was at the woodpile, hacking out stove wood with an axe. When he spied the approaching strange vehicle, he stopped chopping and stared intently. After a few long seconds of staring, he swung the axe downward, wedging the blade into the chopping block for safekeeping, and walked slowly toward the driveway. The white-aproned Miss Ophelia ceased her sweeping activity and was also staring quietly, her left hand propped on her hip.

When he reached the front yard, Mr. Ezekiel's steps quickened, as if he finally realized that the white intruder was probably the cow doctor.

"I'm the cow doctor, Mr. Ezekiel," I yelled, sticking my head out the window. "Where's the cow?"

"She's out here in front of the barn. She's bad sick, white folks!" he replied. It was customary for blacks to address an unknown white person simply as "white folks."

I slowly drove another thirty yards toward the barn, until I could see the downer cow sprawled out in the barnyard. Her baby bull calf, no bigger than a fawn, was lying nearby. He looked bright, alert, dry, and bug-eyed, like Jersey calves are supposed to look. On the other hand, the cow looked bloated and miserable.

As I circled her and thought about what I was going to do, I could see she had already received various treatments in an effort to "cure" her. I was familiar with these home remedies since I had been exposed to them during my internship.

The cow was wearing a strange-looking "bonnet" over her head, and I could see rivulets of blood seeping out from underneath. This meant that someone had already treated her for the "hollerhorn." She smelled strongly of turpentine and kerosene, so I knew that some well-intentioned neighbor who liked to "fool with stock" had dropped by with his "magic potion." There was a raw spot on her loin and a turpentine-saturated corncob on the ground, so I figured that yet another visitor had treated her for the "tightback" by vigorously massaging her spine with the cob.

When I examined her rear parts, I saw that the spot right above her tail switch was neatly wrapped with an old rag and tied in a bowknot. It smelled of black pepper. I wondered if Carney Sam Jenkins had been there, diagnosed "hollertail," and treated her accordingly. It appeared that all the homemade remedies had been tried but the poor patient was still down, unable to rise.

Back at her head, I saw mistletoe leaves and berries scattered about her face and cornmeal smeared prominently on her dry lips. This indicated that someone had tried to poke these substances into her mouth.

Veterinarians or anyone familiar with dairy cows would recognize that Ezekiel and Ophelia's downer cow was suffering from milk fever. Actually, it is misnamed since there is no fever associated with it. It occurs most frequently within seventy-two hours of calving, although it occasionally happens at other times. Basically, it is caused by a deficiency of calcium in the cow's bloodstream. When the calf is born, the cow's udder fills with milk, which is very high in calcium. Sometimes too much calcium is drawn from the blood into the milk and the stage is set for lethargy and even coma. Without treatment, the cow will die.

Injecting calcium intravenously is the treatment of choice and is very effective in most cases, unless there are complicating factors. Often, a cow that is down and out will be standing and apparently normal an hour after treatment. The dramatic response does wonders for a tired vet, weary from too many animal health emergencies and restraining unruly patients.

I rushed to the truck, grabbed a bottle of calcium solution, a needle, and an IV set, and trotted back to the cow. I sat the cow up, punctured the left jugular, and started the warm calcium. As I coiled the tube around her ear, I could hear the familiar "glug, glug, glug" of the solution exiting the bottle and oozing new life into her vein.

"Isn't science great!" I thought to myself, as the cow began to respond minutes later. I could feel her strong heartbeat against my legs as I knelt by her side. When it started to skip a beat every now and then, I pinched the tube and slowed the rate of flow. She was also vigorously beginning to belch off rumen gas, and was becoming aware of her surroundings.

By then Ezekiel was quietly approaching with two foot tubs of water, a bar of lye soap, and an old but clean towel made from a fertilizer sack. I am sure it was the best one they had. Ophelia was standing halfway between the shotgun house and the cow. She was wringing her hands in her apron and praying aloud. I realized then how much their only cow meant to those people.

"What ails her, please sir?" Ezekiel asked shyly. "Is she gonna die?"

"She hasn't got enough calcium in her blood. That's what I'm giving her now," I said.

"I see," he mumbled.

We made small talk as the remainder of the medication slowly dripped into the improving bovine. I removed the needle, then took the equipment back to the truck.

When I returned cowside to wash up, I plunged my hand into the "warm" water, only to discover that it was hot enough to scald hogs. I have found that farmers always bring two-hundred-degree water when you ask for "warm" water. I think it's because they don't know it's hot until it starts to bubble up in the pot. The other tub contained cold spring water, so I alternated between the two and used the lye soap to get my hands clean.

I slipped around behind the cow and bleated like a calf. The old cow's ears perked up and she bellowed throatily. The way she reacted, I knew that she would be standing soon. Sure enough, when I briskly slapped her rump and yelled, she hopped right up and started walking toward Miss Ophelia.

"I knowed this man would fix 'er, Ezekiel! He sho knows about sick cows!"

Ezekiel just stood there slack-jawed, as if he had just witnessed a miracle. While mumbling a series of "yes sirs" and "he sho done its," he busied himself moving buckets and tidying up around the cow's hospital area.

As we all looked proudly at the cow, she started to shake her head and make strange chewing movements. It appeared that she was trying to remove some strange object from her mouth.

Suddenly, she ejected a funny looking "cud." I eased over to where the object was lying on the ground and made a quick examination.

"Why, this looks like an old dishrag soaked with lard," I said in a surprised tone of voice.

"Yes sir," said Ezekiel sheepishly. "I knowed that she had lost her cud, so I put that rag in her mouth, a little while before you got here." He was really embarrassed now. Miss Ophelia was coyly holding her head down and was quietly backing her way toward the storm cellar.

"Well, what you reckon got her up, my medicine or your rag?" I asked, just to see what they'd say.

"Lordy mercy, Doctor," Ophelia declared emphatically, "your medicine done it, your medicine!"

At that point, I think they would have given me the house, the barn, and the mule if I had asked. All I left with, though, was ten dollars, a big bunch of collard greens, two pounds of homemade butter, and a hamper full of sweet potatoes.

I don't think I ever made a more satisfying call.

Chapter 10

THE ALABAMA CATTLEMEN'S Association is a large and powerful organization. Most if not all of Alabama's sixty-seven counties have chapters which meet at periodic intervals, most often about once a month.

The meeting is usually held in the "banquet room" of a local restaurant, in the local school cafeteria, or even a courtroom. Usually a meal is served, which obviously must include some form of beef, most often steak. On rare occasions cattlemen's dinner may replace red meat with fish or chicken, but it will not be well received. During the new-business portion of the meeting, some crusty cattleman can be counted on to stand and lead a team tirade against the wimpy chicken offering and demand that all future dinners include genuine red chewing meat.

Garvis Allen's cafe and motel was not the only eating and sleeping establishment in Butler, but it was the oldest. Located less than one mile south of town, it was a regular stop for many salesmen between Mobile to the south and Tuscaloosa to the north. It was also the place where many locals gathered for meals away from home.

When I arrived at the cafe on a Monday night for my first cattlemen's meeting, I was a little nervous. It was sort of like it was when we attended Butler Methodist Church for the first time, with lots of people staring, trying to figure out who the strangers were.

Nevertheless, I boldly walked in under the big blinking neon EAT sign, past the counter and stools topped with fake red leather, down the single step into the main dining hall, and toward an isolated section way in the back where thirty or forty cattlemen were seated. I knew they were cattlemen because their appearance and demeanor were different from the other patrons'. A couple of them were wearing nice cowboy hats and boots, but most were in clean "farmer" garb. Overalls, flannel shirts, high-top brogan shoes, and seed corn caps were the predominant attire.

That night the cattlemen were sitting around several tables for four and one long table for twelve or so. Their scrambled seating arrangement indicated they were there for camaraderie as well as dining. A few sat astraddle their chairs in backward fashion, leaning their arms on the chair backs, while some had their chairs parked at odd angles away from their tables, happily conversing with their cow-owning comrades a table or two away.

Mr. Rigney, the ag teacher, and Stink Clark waved from a crowded table near the back window. When their eating companions turned, nodded their heads, and smiled, I knew their discussion must be about Stink's bull and the wire that I had removed from his stomach some three days before.

"That's the new vet," I heard someone say. "They claim he's the one that's gonna test all our cows for the Bang's disease."

The federal government, in cooperation with the state department of agriculture, had established a program in Alabama to eradicate Bang's disease from the bovine population. There had been a rumor that Choctaw County was on the list to be tested soon, and after what the farmer said, I suspected that an announcement would be made at the meeting that night.

"Is this seat taken?" I asked two men sitting at a table for four. They were both attired in the standard overalls and flannel shirts. I introduced myself, we shook hands, and I sat down.

"You're just the feller I been wantin' to see," exclaimed the portly one, identified as Jimmy Throckmorton. "I've got this foxhound with a big growth above her upper lip, kind of around to the side of her mouth. Reckon you can put her to sleep and take it off?"

"Yes sir, I'm pretty sure I can."

"Now looka here, boy. This is my finest dog and I want her fixed so you can't tell there was ever nothing wrong with her. I've been offered a thousand dollars for her and I sure don't want anything to happen to her."

"Why don't you bring her down to the house one afternoon and let me look at it, then I can tell you whether or not I can fix it."

"Awright. Don't want no scar or curled-up lip now, you hear? Uh, that won't cost more than ten dollars, will it?"

Mr. Jimmy exemplified one of the things that has always amused me in the practice of veterinary medicine. He wanted Cadillac service for his animals, but he wanted to pay Model T prices.

"Aw, Jimmy, you got plenty money. Doc, don't pay any attention to him, even if he is my brother-in-law and is drawing that big retirement money from the army," exclaimed our dining companion, Mr. Floyd. "And he don't own but one old cow. He came down to this meeting just to see you."

Mr. Sexton walked up about then, along with a smartly dressed, cigar-smoking gentleman.

"Dr. John, this is Dr. Stewart, the federal veterinarian in charge of this area," said Mr. Sexton.

Dr. Stewart was an agreeable Southern gentleman who asked about the health of my family and then expressed optimism about our future in the new town.

"I hope you're ready to go to work because it's gonna be up to you to get this Bang's program rolling after the first of the year. There's about twenty-five thousand cattle in the county, and they've all got to be blood-tested," he declared. "That's going to be a big job, along with the general practice that will come your way."

It certainly would be a "big job" for several reasons.

First, even though it cost the farmers nothing, they had to have all their cows corralled on the arranged date, facilities to handle the cattle, and help to restrain them.

Second, farmers dislike anyone telling them what to do, especially if that person represents the federal government. Therefore, the veterinarian in charge of the testing had to be diplomatic and polite, yet pushy enough to explain the program to the toughest farmer and set up a date for the testing. He could never let on like he was actually a temporary representative of the government.

Third, after the cows were tested, any animals testing positive had to be branded with a "B" and sold immediately. The herd was then quarantined until retested negative twice. Informing a livestock owner that his herd is under quarantine is a difficult task, especially for a young unknown vet, who has not been invited onto the farm in the first place.

"I see. How long do I have to get it done?" I asked.

"Well, you need to get around and get 'em all tested the first time in eighteen months. You do want to do it, don't you?"

"Oh, yes sir. I'm just a little surprised that this is coming along so quickly. But we'll get it done," I replied. It looked like a lot of veterinary work was coming my way!

The meeting started before long, and after the blessing of the meal by Mr. Clyde McDuffie, who was one of the officers, the steaks began to arrive and chatter died down considerably as knives and forks swung into action.

As we ate and conversed quietly, I was surprised at how word of my presence in the county had already spread so quickly. They had heard about Stink Clark's bull eating the wire and they knew about the cows that had eaten too much mash at the Kent Farris farm. They had even heard about the fracas with the snuff choker at the Livingston sale barn.

"Doc, don't take no mess from that Sumter County crowd up at the sale barn. You just come git us if you have any more trouble," one grizzled cowboy declared.

"Yeah, that's right," a few others mumbled. I gathered there was a rivalry between the two counties that had probably started on the high school football field.

Soon the president, Mr. Abston, was introducing the guests, asking us to stand and be recognized. Next came the old-business portion of the meeting which included reports on the big spring rodeo, the calf scramble, and the need to go out and recruit new members. When it came time for new business, he introduced Mr. Sexton.

The extension agent made a few comments about how proud he was to have attracted the first practicing veterinarian to Choctaw County and then he suggested that cattlemen should use the services of that vet when an animal health problem arose.

Next, he introduced Dr. Stewart, who explained that the new Bang's testing program would commence in the county in early 1964 and that every cow would be required to have a blood test. There were some questions and a couple of predictable miniarguments, concerning those people who wouldn't allow the vet to test their cows. Dr. Stewart didn't mince words and suggested that if owners refused to test they could expect to receive a visit from the sheriff or some other high-ranking law enforcement official.

It was probably the most important meeting, from a business stand-point, that I ever attended in my career. Before I left there that night, I talked with many livestock owners who asked for my phone number, several of whom set up appointments for herd work. But no one was more insistent on getting their animals treated than Mr. Jimmy Throckmorton. He was ready to have me operate on old Kate's facial deformity right then, but I prevailed upon him to wait until morning. We decided that since his pen full of dogs needed their rabies shots, worm pills, and heartworm checks, I would just travel to his farm near the town of Robjohn and do the entire job while there for old Kate.

"You want to start early in the morning or on up in the day?" I asked.

"Why don't you just come on about seven o'clock and the wife'll have a bit of breakfast ready. You like sausage?" I nodded. "We just killed hogs, so we've got fresh sausage," he replied.

"Well, if you're sure it won't be too much trouble," I said.

"You gotta eat anyway. So if you don't mind eatin' what we eat, we'd be glad to have you."

My spirits were high as I drove through town on my way home. The events of the evening and the apparent acceptance of the cattle-men again reinforced my belief that we had made the right move.

When I stopped at the traffic light by the post office, the town's policeman was parked over to the side, obviously just waiting for a violator. He quickly blinked his headlights, then flashed on his red light and touched his siren for a second. Since I was the only vehicle in sight, I pulled over and rolled down my window.

"You're Doc McCormack, right?" he said, sternly.

"Oh, no, what is it?" I moaned to myself. "What did I do? I hope some cow owner hasn't sworn out a warrant on me!"

"Yes sir, I am. Is something wrong?"

"Oh no, I'm Walter Kirk, and I've got this dog that's coughing and gaggin' up foam and all. Wonder if he's got worms?"

"Yes sir, Mr. Walter, I wouldn't be a bit surprised. I'll be glad to check him sometime," I declared, trying to sound real professional.

"OK. I could bring him to you up at Mr. Jimmy's tomorrow. That is, if he's around the house that time of the morning."

"At Mr. Jimmy's? How did you know...?"

"I saw him coming through here a while ago and when he stopped to talk he told me about y'all's appointment. He's my cousin, you know."

"Oh, I see."

"Doc, I just keep my eyes and ears open. In a small town like this, I need to know what's going on," he declared. "By the way, we're gonna get some gravel over there on your street this week. Sorry that street's such a mess. You call me if I can ever help, you understand?"

I've often wondered how many veterinarians have been red-lighted and sirened to a stop by friendly policemen who only wanted to ask questions about their sick dogs.

Jan was sitting on the sofa working on an afghan when I arrived home.

"How was your meeting, honey?"

"Great! Had a good steak, met lots of nice folks, and lined up some work," I replied.

"Yeah, I heard about the testing program and all the work you've got to do," she exclaimed.

"What? Where did you hear that?"

"From Mary Lou next door. Her uncle is the president of the Cattlemen's Association and she's also a waitress where y'all met tonight. She heard all about it there. She told me a little while ago when she brought two kittens over here for me to see."

"What? For you to see?"

"Yes, she just wanted to know what sex they were and if they were kin to each other."

"Oh, I see," I said, puzzled.

I was quickly finding out how efficiently a small-town information system works.

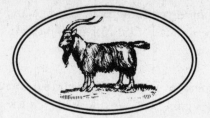

Chapter 11

I THINK EARLY morning is the best time of the day to get out of the house and get work done. You have the road almost to yourself, the air seems fresher and easier to inhale, and the country music station comes in over the airways clearly, which makes the tearjerker tunes twangier and sadder.

Devotees of country music appreciate it for several reasons. The beat and rhythm of these songs are foot-tappingly pleasant, and the sounds that come from the singers' lips are usually recognizable as bona fide words and not some weird-sounding foreign tongue. If you listen carefully to the words and message of a country song it tells a story worthy of careful consideration. Sometimes the lyrics are side-crackingly humorous and tell a true-to-life story, perhaps an incident in the life of any Joe Bob Doe who possesses a pickup truck, has a job, consumes alcoholic beverages, and consorts with members of the opposite sex. If Joe Doe happens to have a wife, carouses a little too much, and gets caught, then he is almost one hundred percent sure to be able to relate, firsthand, to the typical country music song.

Not only do I enjoy country music for the above reasons, but listening to it makes me realize how fortunate I am to have such a loving and understanding spouse and family. It also reminds me to stay out of honky-tonks and avoid all the problems that plague country song writers and singers.

So as I sped northward to Mr. Jimmy's on the newly paved farm-to-market road, I felt good. The clean, brisk November air filled my lungs as the rustic down-to-earth guitar pickin' and singin' made my soul smile. The few vehicles I passed on the road belonged to deer hunters hurrying to their favorite hunting sites, empty pulpwood trucks, and an occasional van load of ladies heading for their jobs at the Vanity Fair plant.

By the time I turned off the main east-to-west road near Robjohn and started up the gravel road, the sun was straining to get above the loblolly pines to the east. I had never paid much attention to pine trees before, but after realizing the dollar value of a load of quality logs or pulpwood, I quickly developed an appreciation for them. The pine tree is a marvelous organism, not only because of its ability to grow quickly in poor soil, but also for the multiple products created from it. It also synthesizes oxygen and provides shade for the sometimes unbearable Southern summer afternoons.

Several pickup trucks and three or so sedans were pulled over to the side of the road as I approached Mr. Jimmy's house. No doubt they had also been invited to breakfast and to watch old Kate's surgery.

The external appearance of Mr. Jimmy's house followed the standard of many of the old Southern country homes of the time owned by folks who scraped a living off the land. Most of these houses were two-story structures, and the standard exterior was clapboard that appeared to detest the thought of a wet paintbrush massage. Even though the building's exterior was lacking in esthetic appeal, its infrastructure was sound, since like most other houses in the fifty- to hundred-year-old class, the studs, sills, and rafters were of solid heart pine. This type of timber would last forever, unless fire, a horrible tornado, or a healthy swarm of hungry termites intervened. Many such houses would ultimately be dismantled and the same pinewood used to reconstruct a grandchild's home just down the road on a piece of Grandpaw's land.

The layout of Mr. Jimmy's house was a little different from most of the country houses I had seen in Choctaw County. As I went up the front steps, I noticed there was no front door in the usual place. Instead, there was a huge ten-foot-wide breezeway separating the first two rooms and continuing out the back as a porch. Through the breezeway, I could see a third room to the right of the porch, with the kitchen situated to the rear of that room. I knew it was the kitchen because of the sounds of laughter and the tinkle of plates and eating utensils being distributed. Presently, Mr. Jimmy appeared at the doorway to the porch.

"Come on in here, boy. Uh, 'scuse me Doc, I ought not be callin' you a boy, but you do look right young," he declared.

"Why, that's a real compliment. But I must be a right smart older than I look," I replied. I had often wished that I looked older, or at least more mature. Older farmers, hunting dog owners, and professional horse trainers had frequently stared at me and wondered aloud if they could trust their valuable and loved animals to my youthful hands.

The kitchen was chock-full of humanity. I counted at least a dozen head of potential diners as they politely eyed the seating arrangements, obviously hoping they would be fortunate enough to land a position at the big table, and not be forced to stand and eat off the counter. Then the table caught my attention.

It was covered with oilcloth and was awash in a sea of traditional breakfast offerings. Steaming platters of meat, eggs, and gravy were being rearranged and moved this way or that in order to create room for more steaming platters of pork chops and grits. I wondered if the four-by-six-foot slab might collapse under such an onslaught of victuals.

"Lord, look at the food!" I exclaimed. "Y'all must have been cooking all night."

"Aw, I just hope it's fittin' to eat," declared one of the three ladies, barely taking time to look up while scanning the area for a suitable site to deposit a newly opened quart jar of homemade pear preserves.

Local tradition and good manners dictated that the above statement be uttered when a visitor made the obligatory compliment on the quantity and esthetic appearance of a set table. In addition to the "I hope it's fit to eat" declaration, there is usually some reference to the insufficiency of the spread. There might be four meats, nine vegetables, three kinds of salad, cathead biscuits, two skillets of cornbread, and a pie safe full of homemade pastries standing by, yet the humble cook would invariably say something like "Aw, it ain't much," or "Well, I just throwed a few things together here," or "If you don't mind eating what we eat, you're more than welcome to what little we've got." These declarations were typical of the time, place, and the station in life that the money-poor but food-rich small farmers then occupied. They possessed few luxury items, but plenty of garden veg-

etables and salt-cured pork were available. Although it might be difficult to justify foxhounds and coonhounds as absolute necessities of life,
hunting dogs were not considered luxury items.

In spite of the large crowd, the country kitchen easily accommo-
dated the oversize rectangular table, all the guests, and the usual appli-
ances and cabinets. There was plenty of walking-around room so that
each cook could work comfortably without constantly colliding with a
pot-handling associate.

Mr. Jimmy's wife was referred to as Miss Dora, and on this day she
was assisted by Miss Julia Fay, who was Miss Dora's older sister and
Mr. Floyd's wife. Then there was a shy teenaged girl, who was the
daughter of the host and hostess, and obviously an apprentice cook.
She mostly handed off skillets and bowls to the more experienced
cooks, and fiddled with used pots in the general vicinity of the sink.

Soon I was seated at the head of the table beside Mr. Jimmy, facing
several unknown neighbors, plus Mr. Floyd, Mr. Kirk from the police
department, and several children.

"Floyd, would you ask the blessin'?" Mr. Jimmy said quietly.

"'Course. Let's bow our heads, please."

I soon found that Mr. Floyd did not believe in being brief when
talking with the Lord. He blessed the crops, the neighbors, prayed for
the sick and afflicted, and asked the Master to give the new veterinary
the skill to heal up all the dogs, and then finally he went into a right
lengthy discussion about the food before us and the fine ladies who
had worked so hard to prepare it.

It was a kind and touching petition, but the aromas from the steaming morsels just inches from my lowered head were cruelly tantalizing
my nostrils as the moments slowly crept by. Finally, it was over and
Mr. Floyd's sincere "Amen" was greeted by our own enthusiastic
"Amens," with our response containing more than a hint of a sigh of
relief.

Plates were quickly loaded with ham, sausage, fried pork chops,
eggs, biscuits, and gravy, and of course, grits. Some say that those individuals who choose to avoid grits are not true Southerners. I vigorously dispute this suggestion, because I was born in the Upper South
and have lived in the Deep South most of my life and I wouldn't place
them anywhere on a list of the top fifty delicious foods. I can and do

eat the ground corn material but I prefer more full-flavored breakfast offerings. Nevertheless, I noticed the breakfast crowd at Mr. Jimmy's had all dipped into the grits bowl with a heavy hand. So heavy, in fact, that Miss Dora had to refill it from a large pot on the stove.

As we ate, Mr. Jimmy introduced all the neighbors, and indicated how many animals each family had. He dwelt upon the canine population, especially the hunting dogs, informing us all as to their pedigrees, their good hunting qualities, and the high intelligence of selected individuals. Occasionally, a neighbor would attempt to speak on behalf of his pen of dogs, but Mr. Jimmy was clearly chairman of this dog-bragging session and he wasn't about to let anyone encroach upon his position of community canine expert.

The dog appreciation seminar continued until syrup-sopping time. As one of the neighbors filled the bottom part of his biscuit-cleaned plate with homemade sorghum syrup, he mercifully changed the subject and made the usual inquiry about the training required for a career in veterinary medicine. My reply was about a one-biscuit-sop answer.

Soon the diners were pushing sopped-clean plates away and were swabbing their mouths with the sleeves of their flannel shirts, in the absence of store-bought napkins. Ladies were swinging into action, removing plates and flatware to the sink, obviously anxious to get on with dishwashing so the next meal could be started and other household chores attacked.

The men donned denim jackets, warmed themselves briefly at the fireplace, and filed out the door toward the dog pen, some placing large chews of tobacco into their cheeks as they went.

Following the recommendation of Mr. Floyd, I carefully backed my station wagon up to the gate of the dog compound and let the tailgate down to use as an examination and surgery table. Perhaps this arrangement wouldn't suit the wishes of every dog owner or veterinarian, but sometimes a makeshift facility is the best you can do.

In order to check the dogs for heartworms, I set the microscope up on the left side of the tailgate and twisted its reflective mirror at just the right angle for the best light. I could then use the right side of the tailgate for my examination table. The dozen or so foxhounds had congregated at the gate, but there wasn't any barking, jumping, or biting at the fence. Instead, all were politely wagging their tails and some were even smiling. I was amazed at their restraint, which was vastly different from the wild antics of deer dogs and coonhounds.

As I injected rabies and distemper vaccines, poked worm pills down their gullets, and drew blood from their large forearm veins, none tried to bite, not even the yearling-aged ones whose stoicism had not yet developed to the level of their more seasoned colleagues. Mr. Jimmy offered tidbits of information about each patient, frequently going into great detail about certain extra-special ones. He elaborated on things like how hard they worked to chase the fox and please their master. The spectators were shaking their heads knowingly as each dog's personal history was briefly reviewed. It was clear that they appreciated dogs, especially good dogs.

I had not paid much attention to the size of the crowd, but toward the end of the clinic I realized that it had grown considerably. Because I was engrossed in my work, I had not heard all the pickup trucks that had filled up the front yard and had pulled over on the shoulders on both sides of the gravel road. Apparently, many in the crowd were passersby who just decided to stop and see what was going on when they saw the crowd.

"Look comin' yonder," someone declared.

"It's old Kate. She's next."

Conversation ceased as Mr. Jimmy proudly led old Kate over to my car and lifted her to the makeshift tailgate examination table. She quietly stood in regal fashion, much to the delight of the audience, while Mr. Jimmy rubbed her hair, checking for ticks, burrs, and other foreign objects, his hands finally coming to rest on a large pus-draining mass on her upper left cheek.

It wasn't really a true mass. It was actually a small opening around which the skin and other tissues had proliferated and then covered over with ugly scabs. A vile discharge was smeared all over the side of her face, which made the problem seem to involve a much larger area than it actually did.

"This thing been on her face very long?" I asked.

"Yes sir, about four months, I reckon," Mr. Jimmy replied. "It kind of swelled up before it busted and started draining."

"Let's get a bucket of water and clean it up. Maybe we can figure this out."

In moments, a fresh pail of well water had been drawn and was presented at my side. A quick scrub with cotton and green soap made the lesion look a lot better, but confirmed my suspicion that the problem came from an infected tooth.

A common dental problem, usually in older, smaller dogs, is an abscessed upper fourth premolar. The tooth has three roots which, when diseased, infect the maxillary sinus. As the infection progresses into the sinus, eventually it ruptures to the outside, creating a draining tract exactly like the one on Kate's face. The tract will continue to drain until the abscessed tooth is extracted, proper drainage established, and antibiotics used.

"What about it, Doc? You ever seen anything like this?" The crowd suddenly grew silent.

"Yes sir, I think I have. I believe it's an abscessed tooth," I replied.

For an instant silence prevailed, until the significance of my diagnosis sunk it. Then the predictable second-guessing began.

"A tooth! Boy, can't you see that thing is on the outside of the dawg?!" exclaimed one expert.

"It's gotta be a wind, I'm tellin' ye!" declared another. Everyone there except the new vet knew that a "wind" (as in "a cold northwest wind") was just a colloquialism referring to a swollen place somewhere on an animal. It might be an abscess, a tumor, or a cyst.

"I 'spec it's cancer," allowed another. "I seen one just like this 'un here on a feller once in the Korean War, and he died!" In his broad Alabama drawl, the disease sounded like "kaon-suh." I could hear other opinions being freely expressed, many of which were weird and bizarre, but very interesting. Finally, Jimmy spoke.

"Is there anything you can do about it?" Conversation once again ceased and quiet descended upon the multitude. The spectators had obviously enjoyed their right to free speech and they were now getting ready to express their differing opinions again when the vet offered his obviously flawed solution.

"Well, we need to put her to sleep, get that tooth out of there, and flush out the abscess," I replied confidently.

This time there were fewer critical remarks, probably because the second-guessers knew less about veterinary surgery than medicine. I did hear a few scattered comments.

"Put 'er t' sleep?! I gotta see that!" one declared. "Reckon he'll use chlorophyll?"

"You mean chloroform," corrected the one who had been in the army. "Naw, he'll probably use ether, 'cause it's a more modern way to put animals to sleep."

"Oh, I see," said the chlorophyll man. He deferred to the wisdom of the war veteran, who had obviously traveled beyond the borders of the county.

"You have to understand that puttin' somethin' to sleep is easy. Wakin' 'em up is what's hard," continued Army. "I was reading a magazine down at Chappell's barbershop just last week and it said that even the use of ether is being phased out now. At the big modern hospitals, they just give patients a shot and it's a lot easier and safer than chloroform or ether."

"Uh huh." It was clear that the boring lecture was getting over the head of Chlorophyll. He didn't care about details. He just wanted to see a dog put to sleep and the operation.

While all the "experts" were delivering their opinions and spattering the bare earth with their used-tobacco expectorant, Mr. Jimmy quietly leaned over and offered a word of welcome advice.

"Doc, don't pay no 'tention to this crowd o' jacklegs. They're all good old boys, but they bump their gums way too much about stuff that they don't know nothin' about. You just go ahead and do what you got to do to fix this dog."

That's what I wanted to hear from the owner of the patient. Now I could get on with it, while paying scant attention to the wild comments of the gallery.

"We'll inject this sodium pentobarbital into her leg vein," I declared purposefully, while drawing about ten cc's of the solution into a glass syringe. There was no sound from the audience except for the stretching of denim galluses as I pointed the needle skyward and expelled exactly one drop of the miraculous, state-of-the-art anesthetic solution. I knew the needle-up, squirt-out-a-drop gimmick would surely get a response, and I wasn't disappointed.

"See what he done just then, Chestuh?" asked a previously unheard-of voice about three standing rows back.

"Huh? What?"

"He squirted a little drop of that sleep dope out 'cause it had some air in it. If he had got that air in that dog's blood veins, she'd have died, graveyard dead before he got the needle out," the voice continued, with a substantial degree of authority. I refused to cut my eyes in that direction, however, for fear of being distracted from my immediate concern.

"Hold her arm vein off like this, Mr. Jimmy," I asked, showing him exactly how I wanted his thumb and fingers to form a temporary tourniquet just above Kate's elbow. With just the right amount of digital pressure, a large and healthy vein swelled and made a promising outline just under the skin. It was an easy chore to quickly slip the sharp needle inside the lumen of the vessel and carefully depress the plunger until Kate slowly collapsed on the tailgate. I checked her toe-pinch and eye-blink reflex continually, injected a few more milligrams, then rechecked again, until she was in a fairly shallow plane of anesthesia. Since extracting the tooth and flushing the sinus was going to be a procedure of short duration, there was no reason for the patient to be deeply anesthetized.

I noticed the doubtful attitude of the crowd was slowly changing into a more positive atmosphere with each movement that I made and with each statement or prediction that I uttered. I realized that I was witnessing a group of individuals who were beginning to show at least an inkling of appreciation for the mysteries of science and medicine.

The problem with extracting the tooth was its deep three-root system. Perhaps such an anatomical arrangement is easy pickings for my human dentist colleagues, but the training that veterinarians received in animal dentistry in the 1950s was somewhat superficial. Now, some thirty-five to forty years later, the study of canine and feline dentistry receives a great deal of attention in veterinary school.

I knew that in order to remove the tooth without fracturing one of the roots, it would be necessary to split the tooth in half to remove first one half, then the other. I slipped on a pair of rubber gloves and quickly elevated the gum line. Then, with a steel pin and chuck, I drilled a hole from the cheek side to the tongue side of the tooth. This done, I retrieved a foot-and-a-half length of embryotomy wire from my black bag.

Embryotomy or Gigli wire is composed of several rough, sharp strands of small-diameter wire, which, when woven together tightly, make an ideal and inexpensive instrument for sawing through bone, hoof, horn, and even tooth.

The crowd was inching closer and closer to the gum line action and when I threaded the wire through the small hole, two grimy hands appeared out of the mass of humanity and attempted to pick up the elusive end as it poked through.

"Uh, uh! Don't touch it!" I yelled. "Are those hands clean?"

Both hands snapped back into overall pockets like cuckoos back into their clocks. They obviously wanted so much to be a part of Kate's healing process they never considered the fact that rusty, filthy hands might set up more infection in the dog's highly inflamed gums.

With a pair of forceps, I fished the loose end of the wire out of the hole, attached a handle on to each end, and started quick to-and-fro sawing motions.

"Y'all hold her head real steady now, whoever's got the cleanest hands," I declared.

While two sets of pale, obviously "downtown" hands secured Kate's head, I continued the sawing motion, going faster and faster until smoke and minute tooth particles lightly puffed into the air with every stroke. After no more than a minute, the cut was complete and the tooth was divided into two equal parts. Then, using my secondhand army surplus molar extractor, I latched on to the rear half of the tooth. With firm traction and a series of half twists, the single-rooted rear portion eased out of its tight resting place. I dropped it into the bottom of an awaiting metal bucket with a resounding "plink," just like I had seen those Western shoot-em-up town doctors do on TV. The crowd was duly impressed.

I knew the other half was going to present a more stubborn pull and I so informed the spectators. They were getting into this surgery thing, and I was almost engulfed by assistants and Kate's admirers to such a degree that I was in danger of being jostled back into the second row. But using the perseverance of an Auburn football fan, I doggedly stood my ground and maintained my rightful place as dog dentist of the hour.

Now with several assistants holding on, I secured my army instrument to the remaining tooth remnant and began the extracting movements. However, this time nothing was budging, even though I could see a portion of what I thought was root, bone, or strange foreign body wiggling around up on the side of Kate's face, inside the mass. So when I had no success below, I directed my attention higher up on the cheekbone in the area of the moving mass and began to probe around with a pair of forceps.

Things began to happen. Manipulating the forceps resulted in several necrotic pieces of cheekbone becoming detached and falling to the ground, much to the delight of the crowd, many whom were quickly becoming board-certified dental surgeons, at least in their own minds.

More and larger pieces of bony debris loosened and fell away as I swabbed the area with gauze sponges. Soon I realized that I was staring down into the maxillary sinus and directly at the diseased root of the tooth. Suddenly, I heard a suggestion offered from a couple of rows back.

"'Scuse me Doc, but I was just thinkin' about somethin'," said a gruff voice. "I'm a riveter down at the shipyard in Mobile and I was wonderin' if it'd work better if you punched that snag out from the top, 'stead of tryin' to pull it out the bottom?" For all the cockeyed analysis I had heard from the spectators, I had to admit this was a pretty good idea.

"Uh, yeah, that might work, except I don't have a punch or a hammer," I replied.

Immediately, a brace of denim-clad bodies dashed to their beloved pickup trucks, grabbed their beloved toolboxes out of the back, then raced back and placed the implements at my feet.

"Nothing, not even their Craftsmen tools, is too good for old Kate," I joked to myself, while staring at the vast assortment of punches available for my use. "I just hope my surgery professor doesn't hear about this."

Kate had been sleeping soundly and her breathing was regular and deep, but now she was reacting to the toe-pinch and eye-blink reflex, so I knew I needed to finish up the job in short order.

I quickly selected a bright, almost new punch, sloshed it around in some Roccal disinfectant that I had poured into the bottom of a pail, and leveled the working end of it on the outside part of the tooth root.

"OK now, one of y'all take that hammer and give me a few taps on this punch," I requested.

After a few blows I felt the root collapse down through its resting place in the jaw. Then a few taps on the inside portion of the root resulted in its also falling out onto the tailgate. I quickly packed the gaping cavity in the bone with gauze sponges to temporarily stop some of the blood flow. I would deal with that presently when I diverted the attention of the audience to something else.

"Y'all look at the rotten spots on these fragments," I declared. "Can't you imagine the toothache she must have had!"

As the tooth parts passed from hand to hand, each amateur dentist carefully examined and fondled them before issuing his opinion on how long and how severe Kate's pain had been. While they were thus entertained, I extracted the gauze and explored the diseased gum, sinus, and bone, while removing necrotic debris. After cleaning it up nicely, I saturated a long strip of three-inch gauze with an antibiotic, folded it on itself two or three times, then inserted it up into the cavity through the maxillary sinus, finally forcing it out the opening on the side of her face. A strip of gauze used in such a manner is called a "seton," and it keeps an infected cavity open for drainage.

Next, I drew up a dose of penicillin with needle and syringe, pointed the needle toward the heavens, thumped the side of the syringe with my forefinger, then carefully squeezed out one drop, just like I had done before, and injected it into Kate's leg.

"Wow! Did you see how quick he give that shot?" I heard someone exclaim. "I wish them real doctors down at Butler was that fast!"

"Aw, ain't nothin' to it," another voice declared. "Jus' like stickin' a pin in a cantaloupe. I coulda' done nat!"

I just smiled.

Minutes later, we had Kate bedded down in the corner of the corn-crib on a deep blanket of pine straw. She was beginning the slow awakening process, moving her legs and occasionally licking her lips.

With the work completed, the spectators were heading for their trucks in twos and threes, some still conversing animatedly, no doubt expounding upon their theories as to how the surgery they had just observed could have been done better. In just seconds, most of the trucks had departed, leaving a great cloud of dust permeating the house and yard.

As Mr. Jimmy and I washed up instruments and other paraphernalia at the well in the yard, one of his daughters came out of the kitchen door and paused at the steps.

"Daddy, Momma said to tell you she's got some tea cakes and coffee for you and the veterinary if y'all want it," she announced.

"Awright, we'll be there in a minute," he replied.

It was only midmorning and only hours before we had feasted on a breakfast fit for royalty! More food that soon was the last thing I wanted or needed! However, I knew that I could not refuse the hospitality of such sincere and thoughtful people.

"Maybe I'll eat just one little cookie and half a cup of coffee as Mr. Jimmy and I discuss Kate's aftercare," I thought to myself.

Twenty minutes later, I was happily biting into my fourth colossal cookie. Miss Dora's offerings were at least four inches in diameter and their tops were smeared with fudge.

"I'll declare, Miss Dora, these things are superb! They're just like the ones my grandmama used to bake for me," I mumbled, talking with my mouth full in a way Grandmama would've frowned on.

"Aw, I just throwed 'em together. Hope they're fit to eat," she answered, while stirring something cooking in a big pot on the stove.

I stopped by Mr. Jimmy's while making rounds over the next several weeks. Kate's wound healed nicely and she hunted several more years, much to the pleasure of all the foxhunters in southwest Alabama and east Mississippi. And since the Kate episode was so widely discussed where foxes were run and tales told, it gave me an instant reputation as a "pretty good dog doctor." From then on, it was common practice to see a pickup truck loaded with foxhounds pull up in front of my house.

In addition, my education in becoming a country veterinarian continued that day at Mr. Jimmy and Miss Dora's. First, I was learning how to handle, if not to enjoy, the second-guessing of owners and spectators. Country veterinarians, by necessity, perform difficult and challenging barnyard surgery under the critical eye of any Joe Bob, Buck, or Bubba who happens to be passing along the road at that time and decides to stop. There are no secrets vets can hide from wide-eyed viewers since they aren't behind closed doors or a KEEP OUT sign. And in this case, the crowd had even supplied some of the surgical instruments, so I could hardly complain.

Second, I was learning more and more about the strength of the bond between humans and their pet companions. That association was unlike the economic bond between a farmer and his livestock. If a cow or pig didn't provide a financial payoff in some way, that animal was a liability to the operation, and it was invited on a one-way trip to town. But even the most practical folks would go to great lengths to get a favorite pet cared for.

Third, I was learning that most people treat their veterinarian as a special person, and frequently have refreshments prepared when he or she is on the premises.

When I was a lad, my momma tried hard to teach me proper manners and etiquette. I am sure she wondered many times if all those efforts had been in vain. Perhaps that is the reason I feel obliged to accept those offers of farm buffet breakfasts, tea cake breaks, and tall glasses of cold iced tea. I wouldn't want to disappoint Momma. It's just a burden I'll have to bear.

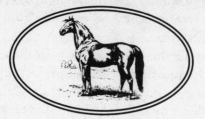

Chapter 12

A COUPLE OF weeks passed and I was happily surprised at how busy I was so early in the new practice. Dealing with the homemade veterinarians had not yet been a significant problem, but on many calls the name of Carney Sam Jenkins had been used in reverence. It was apparent that his dirt-road brand of animal medicine had set the standard for other would-be veterinarians who practiced part-time in the Choctaw County area. I was not looking forward to it, but knew it was time to pay him a visit.

I was afraid there was going to be some ill will between the two of us. It was likely that he was going to lose some income because of the new vet in the county as well as his status as the foremost animal health authority in the area. On the other hand, I felt he should not be practicing veterinary medicine without a license. Since he possessed no license and had no government accreditation, any veterinary treatment he performed for a fee was against the state practice act.

I remembered what Mr. Sexton had said about Carney Sam when I visited him in his office right after I arrived in Butler. He was trying to tell me that if I avoided a confrontation with Carney Sam things would go a lot better for me in the community. Lecturing him about his illegal activities would do nothing but antagonize him as well as his friends. All I had to do was swallow a large dose of new-graduate pride and try to work with him, if he would allow it. The hard part would be trying to keep my lip zipped when faced with some of his tail-splitting treatments. But I knew the diplomatic way was the only way to survive in Choctaw County.

I found out that Carney spent a portion of every morning at Miss

Ruby McCord's country store and service station near his house. Her store was located on a farm-to-market road that I had already traveled several times. It was conveniently situated at an intersection and had many beckoning signs erected, which no doubt caused many a traveler to stop in for a cold drink and a candy bar.

The country store was the nerve center of a rural area. It was a place for socializing and hearing all the latest rumors, as well as picking up groceries and supplies. Frequently it was the site of the only telephone in the community and the storekeeper often had to make the calls since some folks were still uncomfortable with the contraption.

Since her store was on my way to the sale barn, I decided to drop by there on a Thursday morning and ask Carney Sam to accompany me to the sale that day. That would give us an opportunity to hold our conference in the privacy of my car rather than in the store in front of the customers.

The next Thursday morning, as I arrived at Miss Ruby's store, I observed a rusty, old, doorless International pickup truck backed halfway up on a large mound of red clay. My past experience with clunker cars and junker trucks told me that the truck was up on the mound because it had a balky battery and was waiting for a roll start. I knew the rusty truck belonged to Carney Sam because I could see needles, syringes, and a couple of small bottles of cow medicine atop the instrument panel.

There were other parked vehicles—an old car, a farm wagon hitched to a team of blue-nosed mules, and a Colonial Bread truck. In the bushes off to the side I saw at least two junk cars up on blocks, obviously long since retired, whose usable parts had been cannibalized and relocated to other vehicles in ill health. This transferring of parts accounted for the preponderance of white cars with black fenders and Ford sedans dressed with hubcaps of Buick or Plymouth origins.

From inside the store came the sound of masculine voices punctuated by sporadic laughter. I detected an occasional audible word, such as "idiots," "stupidity," and "leeches," so I knew from previous similar experiences that the present conversation was about "the govmunt."

"The govmunt" was a phrase always spoken in a quick, disgusted tone of voice, as if the word caused a horrible taste on the base of the tongue and had to be spit out as quickly and as curtly as possible. This term referred only to the federal government that was "up yonder" in

Washington, not the state or local government. Any passing car with a sticker or painted logo on its door was assumed to be occupied by a "govmunt leech" and was thus to be viewed with contempt and avoided if at all possible. Exceptions could be made for the soil-conservation man since he helped to build pasture ponds and he usually drove a pickup truck, which elevated him a notch or two on the government-leech scale.

I hesitated briefly at the screen door because I hated to interrupt the government-bashing colloquium. Breaking into their proceedings when they were all fired up and mad could be hazardous to my well-being. If they knew that the government was paying me to test cows at the sale barn, they might vent their anger in my direction. And I didn't have a pickup truck yet.

Drawing up to my full six feet, I grabbed the screen door handle, the one that proclaimed COLONIAL IS *GOOD* BREAD, pushed the old wooden door open, and stepped inside. For about three seconds there was complete silence as several sets of eyes riveted their stern stares on the unknown intruder.

"Mornin', how're y'all," I exclaimed, trying hard to produce a tough-looking smile in front of clenched teeth.

A few heads nodded a silent greeting while one, apparently the sitter with the most seniority, offered the only verbal response.

"Awright, but just a mite nippy, ain't it," he allowed. As he spoke, the assistant and young apprentice store sitters peered at him respectfully.

I counted four sitters arranged in a semicircle around the stove. They sat on nail kegs and mineral blocks, occasionally spitting with perfection into a topless three-pound coffee can at the base of the stove. An elderly lady stood behind the counter scribbling entries in a ledger book. The Colonial man was stalking around the bread rack fiddling with the loaves, rearranging them or just moving them forward or backward an inch or two.

Country store sitters are not viewed as necessities of life, but their presence does add much to the quality of life out in rural areas where the pace is a lot slower and the television choice is limited to one channel. Sitters simply know everything, and don't mind informing anybody who will listen. They keep up with all the news relating to local politics, mortuary admissions, school news, crop reports, marital disharmony, weather predictions, and, of course, college football.

The sitter who had responded to my greeting seemed to be the head sitter. There was an aura of authority around him and he was older than the others, plus he had the best-looking nail keg. He presented a certain toughness as he sat there, whittling and spitting. He was about five feet ten inches tall and was chunky but not fat. With short, muscular arms and a wide body, he reminded me of someone who would have made a pretty good guard on the football team had he been available for the opportunity.

He wore a red-checkered flannel shirt, Washington Dee Cee bib overalls, and black engineer's boots, which were of black leather with a little chrome buckle at the top, just below the knee. His red cap proudly advertised Funk's G Hybrid seed corn. He talked curtly and gruffly. I knew he must be Carney Sam.

"I'm Dr. McCormack, the new veterinarian," I declared.

"Jenkins. Carney Sam Jenkins," the older one replied. "Are you gettin' any business yet?" The other sitters said nothing, but continued to stare.

"Yes sir, I'm getting more calls than I anticipated. There seems to be plenty of vet work around here."

"Yeah, me too. They just won't leave me alone, Doc. Ever' night somebody's out front of the house mashin' on their horn or hollerin' for me to come out and mess with somethin' sick."

The silent sitters were scrutinizing me carefully. I knew they were committing every detail of my appearance and demeanor to their memory, so they could report to ensuing customers and family members that they had seen, firsthand, the new veterinarian.

More polite talk ensued, covering the weather, who was killing hogs that day, the condition of cows, and the high price of veterinary service. One of the associate sitters made a remark every now and then, but it eventually turned into a question-and-answer session. They were asking the questions and I was trying to formulate answers.

"Tell me this, vetran," one of the bolder sitters asked. "Did you have to go to some kind of school to learn how to doctor on stock or did you just take it up?"

"Yeah, I went to seven years of college before I got my degree and passed the exam to get my license," I replied, as I had done many times before.

"*Seven years!*" the sitters all exclaimed in unison. All except Carney Sam, who was quietly filling his old corncob pipe with tobacco out of a Prince Albert can.

"Why didn't you go on to school a little longer and be a real doctor?" was the easily predicted question that followed.

"Because I don't like fooling with people!" I allowed, real serious-like.

After a few seconds I grinned and they started to laugh. That seemed to break the ice, and Carney Sam spoke again.

"Being a vet is a lot more than knowin' how to doctor on stock. You better have a sense of humor to go along with it, if you want to be able to enjoy yourself while you're livin' your life," Carney Sam declared.

"That's right, that's right!" all the sitters echoed.

"Doc, you in a big hurry?" Carney Sam suddenly exclaimed.

"No, but I need to be at the sale barn about noontime," I replied.

"How 'bout runnin' up to the house with me? I want to show you somethin'."

"Sure, I've got a couple of hours to spare. I'll follow you in my car," I replied.

I was somewhat taken aback by the invitation to visit his home. Now my plan of a station wagon conference with him seemed unlikely.

Carney Sam's place was less than a half mile from Miss Ruby's store. When we neared the proper turnoff, Carney simply eased over onto the left side of the road, slowed down, and negotiated a tight left turn between an unmarked, leaning mailbox and a large pine tree.

I had noticed that most rural people in Choctaw County did not have their names or any other sort of identification on their mailboxes. It made it more difficult for me to locate clients who had called for veterinary service.

"Why don't y'all have your names on your mailboxes?" I asked a group of watchers one day while dehorning calves.

"Well, so won't nobody know where we live at!" explained one.

"Why don't you want anybody to know where you live?" I asked, puzzled.

"Why would we want 'em to know?" was the answer. "Anybody

that's comin' to see us already knows where we live." The group looked at me like I needed my brain audited.

Later I realized there was a certain logic to their attitude. Most of the folks you'd want to see had probably lived in the area since birth. So why make it easier for strangers, who were probably salesmen, revenuers, or govmunt leeches, to find you?

As my vehicle rattled up to the house, three curs came hurtling out from the wide-open spaces underneath the house as if the Communists had arrived. The hair along the center line of their backs was standing straight up and their slobbery snarling and barking was loud enough to disturb the dead. It was apparent that they were all suffering from some highly irritating form of dermatitis, probably fleas or red mange, because every few steps a dog would pause, sit for a few seconds, and enthusiastically scratch some portion of his or her anatomy with a hind leg. The antics and the dermatological problems of his dogs caused me to wonder about Carney Sam's level of expertise on the canine species. I knew they served no economic purpose, other than doing away with table scraps and trying to scare off strangers, but I wondered if the level of veterinary service he delivered to the pets of his clients was as inadequate as what I observed in his own dogs. Perhaps he was so busy treating the pets of others he had no time for his own.

Carney's old smoking jalopy sputtered and jerked to a stop out behind the house, just in front of a small, twenty-foot-square concrete block structure. It appeared to have been constructed by someone totally lacking in building skills. Nothing about it appeared level, the blocks protruded in various places, and there were large gaps between the door and the frame. Just above the door the word TAXIDERMIST was lettered unevenly in black paint.

"Nice building!" I yelled, trying to be heard above the dog racket. I was staring at the building in disbelief and wondering why I had just lied.

"Yeah I think so, built it myself," he replied. *"Shut up!"*

Immediately all the dogs silently tucked their tails and cowered their way back under the house, licking their lips, grinning, and holding their heads down at various angles.

Inside the building, Carney led me to a corner where there were a small table, a shelf of drugs, and two cages. I assumed this was the vet department. Inside one cage was a small terrier dog with her new puppies. She appeared to be in distress.

"Doc, what do you think ails this dog? She's feverish, real excitable, pantin' hard, and looks like she's about to go into a spasm."

"How long has she been like this?" I asked, looking closer. A strong odor of turpentine and Mr. Kent Farris's moonshine liquor rose from the cage.

"A lady brought her in from over yonder in Mississippi early this morning. She said she started actin' kind of strange in the middle of the night. I believe she's either poisoned or got the kidneyitis," he declared. "Said this was her little girl's dog and if anything happens to this dog, it'll just kill that child. They left here goin' to town, but they'll be back by here directly. What chu reckon it is, Doc?"

I didn't want to get into a discussion on this "kidneyitis" thing that he mentioned. I would find out later that his favorite diagnosis in dogs was "kidneyitis." But if he didn't think kidneyitis was the problem, then he would diagnose poisoning.

The dog with the puppies appeared to be suffering from eclampsia, which is an acute deficiency of calcium occurring in dogs that have recently had puppies. It is essentially the same condition that affected Ezekiel and Ophelia's cow but the symptoms are quite different. Affected cows are down and almost comatose, while dogs are usually feverish and highly excited.

"She's got eclampsia, Carney. Are you familiar with that?"

"Uh, seems like I might have read something about that some-where," he answered. I wondered if reading was difficult for him, especially that of a scientific or medical nature. When he was a boy, he likely completed three or four grades of grammar school and that was considered adequate, but fifty or so years later that thinking would prove to have been a mistake. In the 1960s others like Carney could sign their names and negotiate simple newspaper articles, but trying to understand something as complicated as medical textbooks with all those big, foreign-type words was difficult, so most just avoided such attempts.

I hurried to my car, picked up a needle, syringe, and a bottle of cal-cium gluconate. I filled the syringe as I walked back inside the dual vet clinic/taxidermy shop.

"What a combination," I thought to myself. "My classmates and vet school professors wouldn't believe it!" If they found out that such a combination existed, they would be shocked and appalled. I could just hear the ageless, articulate, and purse-lipped professor of veterinary surgery and obstetrics and chairman of the ethical standards committee ranting and raving.

"The noble practice of veterinary medicine cannot be adulterated by the addition or merging of other vocations, such as taxidermy. This would be the equivalent of an M.D. practicing in a funeral parlor. Our professional creed and code of ethics precludes such activity and behavior."

Perhaps some of those ivory-towered professors should have gone out into the real world to find out what was really happening in the country. Sometimes things aren't always as black and white out there as they are sitting behind a desk in a nice comfortable office.

Carney had the little ten-pound black-and-white mixed breed dog out of her cage and semirestrained on the old rickety table when I returned from the car.

"Hold her tight, Carney. This has got to go in her leg vein, and the way she's shaking it may be hard to hit." I sure didn't want to have trouble with this vein, especially with the county's number-one homemade veterinarian looking on.

With a tourniquet at elbow level, I carefully palpated the vessel. It wasn't large, but it stood up nicely, probably because of her excited condition.

"Lord, I don't ask for much. But just this once, I hope you'll see fit to help me get this needle placed in this blood vein," I prayed, or something to that effect. I don't believe in asking for special favors, since I know the Master has problems more pressing than helping a nervous country veterinarian give dog injections. But I felt like this was an unusual case.

"You got it, Doc! You got it!" exclaimed Carney Sam as the needle slipped easily into the vein and blood flowed back into the syringe. Who said the Master didn't answer prayers?

"Shh, shh, be real quiet," I cautioned. "Don't want her getting upset." I slowly injected the calcium into the vein, a little at a time. If the calcium goes too fast, two things can happen. First, the dog may vomit, which isn't too bad. Second, the calcium may cause the heart to stop—which is real, real bad.

Some five or so minutes later, the last drop of medicine had been forced into the bloodstream. Now we had to wait a few minutes to see the outcome. As we placed the dog back in the cage, I noticed that she was already less jumpy and her panting had dropped a notch or two. I could also see a big difference in Carney's attitude. It was like he was beginning to accept me as an animal doctor and as a person.

"Doc, I'm impressed. You sure knew how to get that vein," Carney allowed. "I have trouble with those little veins. My eyes are bad, you know, on account of the Bang's disease I got from cleaning off cows years ago. I usually just give 'em something by mouth."

"Well, what was that odor I smelled? Was it whiskey?" I asked.

"Uh, yeah it was." He grinned sheepishly. "I wasn't sure what ailed her, but I knew if it was kidneyitis or poison, then some homemade liquor would put her plum right, you know. So I just gave her a dram or two just in case." He quickly changed the subject and pointed over to the other side of the room, where there were several mounted deer heads, a few fish on plaques, and tanned hides hanging on the wall.

"Looka here, Doc, at these deer heads. And this bobcat I just finished mountin' for a feller over in Georgia. Ain't he a beauty?"

His taxidermy was first class and it was obvious that he took much pride in what he did. But it was clear he was not nearly as skilled a veterinarian as he was a taxidermist. His diagnosis was rudimentary, and his treatment—drenching a critically ill canine with white lightning whiskey—was inappropriate.

Now he was into giving me advice, filling me in on all the hunt clubs and the status of deer and turkey populations in the county.

"You need to get your name on the Rudder Hill Hunting Club waiting list right away," he declared. "The hunting is good and all the big shots belong."

Then he named the leading fox and coon hunters in the area, and suggested where I should go fishing. Next, he advised which county citizens wouldn't pay their bills, and he let me in on how all the rich people had come into their money. It was a valuable and eye-opening seminar.

As we made our way back over to the veterinary side of the business, the little dog that had been so sick just twenty minutes before was now standing at the cage door, wagging her tail.

"Why it's a miracle," Carney yelled, with both hands above his head. "It's a plum miracle!"

While he was going on about the dog and talking to her through the door, we heard a car pull up outside, and presently there were several light taps on the door. A young woman in her late twenties peeked around the door.

"I just thought I'd come back to see if my little girl's dog is any better," she said quietly. "She's really all tore up about it. You know, we got her that dog on account of her asthma."

"Yes ma'am, I understand." Carney was opening the cage door and the dog made a beeline to the lady, yapping and trying to jump up her legs.

"Why, it's a miracle," she exclaimed. "Just hours ago she was at death's door! It's a plum miracle!"

Looking out the window, I could see the sad face and red eyes of the little girl of six or seven sitting alone in the old car. I'm sure she had given up the thought of ever seeing the dog alive again.

While the lady hand-carried the patient out to the car, Carney was carefully depositing her puppies in a nice towel-lined cardboard box. I watched through the window, realizing that I was momentarily going to observe one of the most pleasurable sights veterinarians can enjoy.

When child and dog spied each other, it was hard to tell which was the happiest. The long tear-stained face in the car instantly became a picture of jubilation. The dog was wiggling all over, and her tail and hind end were going from side to side a hundred times a minute. Now the dog was almost up in the girl's face, trying to lick, trying to yap, trying to climb higher. It was only a dog, but the happiness created by that dog could not be assessed by any tangible measuring device.

"This is the smart man who saved your dog," Carney Sam told the lady. "He's our veterinarian for the county, and he's gonna build a fine clinic down at Butler. I recommend him highly."

I was dumbfounded to hear him give me the credit for saving the dog. As the lady shook my hand and offered multiple thanks, I was thinking about what Carney Sam had said. "Fine clinic," "smart," "recommend him highly." What did all this mean?

As the satisfied clients drove slowly back down the hill, I felt good. Perhaps we had accomplished two things. We had saved a dog from certain death, and Carney and I had gotten together.

"Doc, you know I can't quit doin' a little vet work, 'cause folks won't leave me alone and I just can't tell 'em no. But I'm gonna do all I can to help you. I saw the way you looked at that little girl and her dog, and I know you like to help folks. And I believe you know your business." He stuck out a formaldehyde-hardened hand and we shook hands for the first time. I was learning more and more about how diplomacy and tact make the world go around. Despite my flippant comment to the store sitters, this morning's experience showed that, medical knowledge aside, being skillful with people is a necessity for success as a veterinarian.

The ride back down the driveway seemed a lot more pleasant than coming in, even though the three dogs got a head start on me this time. They were biting at the tires and one was running on ahead of me, as if he was going to head me off at the main road.

About halfway down the hill, I heard Carney yell at the top of his voice.

"Shut up!"

Instantly, the curs stopped, hushed, and disappeared back into the trees.

"It's a miracle." I laughed. "It's a plum miracle!"

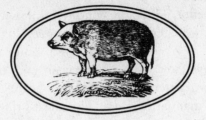

Chapter 13

"DOC, WE GOT a cow that needs to be cleaned off. Can you come out?"

Unless you are a veterinarian, cow owner, or someone who "fools with stock," this request can be quite confusing. Upon listening to such an utterance, some of my livestock-illiterate friends and acquaintances can be observed furrow-browed and tilt-headed, trying to figure out its meaning.

I'll admit that the expression "cleaning off a cow" could be improved upon. In fact, a more appropriate approach would be to ask the veterinarian to clean *out* a cow. I will now, in an effort to advance the cause of veterinary internal medicine, attempt to clear up the "clean off a cow" business, realizing that some will say it is not exactly proper for living room discussion. Those individuals with sensitive systems might want to skip the next few paragraphs.

Even novice students of the bovine species are acutely aware that these four-legged creatures are different from other quadrupeds. Cows have no upper teeth, except for molars, and they have a weird arrangement of four stomachs, which enables them to consume all sorts of hays, grasses, and otherwise high-cellulose byproducts. The fact that they can convert these forages into milk and meat is in itself a miracle of nature. In addition to possessing a complex digestive tract, their reproductive system is also different. The cow's placenta, which is the membrane system that covers and nourishes the fetus, is attached to the uterus through a series of large buttonlike structures called caruncles.

Occasionally, after the birth of the calf, the placenta is not expelled as intended by nature. Instead, due to reasons of nutrition, stress, or environment, the little buttonlike caruncles maintain their tight connection to the placenta. Thus, the condition known as "retained placenta" occurs, and the veterinarian is summoned to clean off the cow.

The call may be received as early as a few hours after calving, or it may be several days later. The veterinarian may treat the problem with injectable or intrauterine medications, but the older, more traditional treatment is manual removal. This means that a hand and arm must be introduced up into the cow's reproductive tract, and the membranes manipulated loose from their attachments. It is not the most pleasant of tasks.

But this is only the beginning. Imagine a fifteen-pound mass of rotten membranes hanging down two to three feet from the rear parts of the patient. Each day the mass hangs there without any hope of being expelled, the more putrid the thing becomes and the farther away it can be smelled. There are no words to describe the smell of a five-day-old retained placenta, still attached deep in the innards of the cow, in the hot July or August weather of west Alabama.

My first such case in Choctaw County was not long in coming. Jan took the call while I was out on a night visit.

"Mr. C. Y. Turner down at Gilbertown called and wants you to clean off a cow," Jan said when I arrived home. "I told him you'd be there the first thing in the morning. The directions are there by the phone."

I have always thought that it is important for a practicing veterinarian to have a caring and understanding spouse. That spouse must understand that veterinary medicine is a service profession and unless it responds to the needs of the animal-owning public, the practice will not be successful. A spouse must also be aware of the importance of a good telephone manner and the absolute necessity of obtaining good directions when arranging for a farm call. This may seem like a small concern, but farmers are notorious about giving out poor directions, and a vet who can't find the patient in the first place is unlikely to have a high success rate.

Fortunately for me, Jan has no equal in the ability to get detailed directions to a farm. Her concerned and friendly attitude always puts worried callers at ease.

The next morning around seven-thirty found me easily finding Mr. C. Y.'s farm and encountering the first of two gaps. Let it now be documented that I am a world authority on gaps. Instead of an expensive store-bought gate, nearly every small-acreage farmer that I have ever known makes a homemade gate by stringing three or four strands of barbed wire from a strong corner post over to a movable, smaller post some six to ten feet away, depending on the width of the opening to be protected. When closed, the bottom of the movable post is secured by dropping it into an oversized loop of baling wire around the bottom of the second corner post. When the gap is stretched taut, a second over-sized loop of baling wire circles the top of both posts. There are several variations on this arrangement, depending upon geographical locale and farmer ingenuity.

Back then in Alabama and Tennessee, it was not uncommon to pass through one of these gaps, or even a series of them, before reaching the barn, back pasture, or corral. The constant getting out of the vehicle, letting down the gap, getting back in the vehicle, driving through the opened gap, getting back out, putting up the gap, getting back in the vehicle, and driving toward yet another gap was almost enough to send a busy veterinarian running wildly toward the kudzu, screaming and strumming his lower lip with his shaking fingers.

When I reached the second gap just in front of the house and some fifty yards downwind from the barn, I caught a whiff of the reason for my visit. I couldn't detect the exact source of the terrible odor, but my intuition told me it was coming from the direction of the dilapidated barn.

Actually, there were several outbuildings, which was typical of a Southern barnyard. The centerpiece was, naturally, the main barn. It was sort of like the administration building on a college campus, but without the clock or tower. The typical barn in that area was old, unpainted, and had a minimum of two mule stalls, a corncrib, spacious hayloft, and a tack room of sorts. In addition, there was usually some sort of lean-to shed off one side or the other, which was used to keep worn-out mule-drawn cotton planters and turning plows from complete deterioration. The signature room was the main hallway, wide enough to accommodate hay wagons and mule dewormings.

Some barnyard compounds contained a pole barn, which was made from stout cedar, locust, or perhaps poplar tree trunks. A few rafters made from scrap lumber were nailed up and this topped with scavenged tin. This barn was used to store baled hay, wagons, and any other type of equipment that needed a roof overhead. There was an outdoor toilet on the periphery and frequently a mystery building, similar to a small corncrib, which was used for numerous purposes, including housing female dogs when they came into heat. All honorable farmers attempted to pen up their female dogs when they went through this trying time, even though male dogs can dig under, gnaw through, or climb over almost any device created by man.

As I rehung the second gap, Mr. C. Y. came limping out of the side door. He had obviously waited until I came through the gap before he showed himself. No need of straining himself to open gaps for that young whippersnapper veterinarian, I'm sure he was thinking.

I never knew why Mr. C. Y. limped. There were so many lame farmers all over the area that it didn't even register on me after a while. It seemed that a lot of these people had worked in the timber industry earlier in their careers so I always figured that trees had fallen on them and smashed their legs or hips. Or perhaps it was because they were always getting kicked and stepped on by unruly cows and horses. Sometimes because medical care was not readily available or cost money farmers didn't have, fractures healed improperly or not at all, resulting in permanent crippling.

After we exchanged pleasantries, Mr. C. Y. indicated that the cow was in one of the mule stalls. While he windlassed up a bucket of water from the shallow well, I retrieved a shoulder-length rubber obstetrical sleeve, rope, disinfectant soap, and my medical bag from the back of the car. Soon we were trudging toward the barn, each carrying an armload of veterinary equipment.

I had already learned that at least three very important things could be accomplished while walking with the farmer to the barn or wherever the patient was located. First, I always tried to obtain a short history of the patient and her illness. I asked about her appetite, her attitude, bowel activity, level of milk production, duration of illness, change in feeding patterns, and whether there had been any previous treatments.

Taking a short history often proves impossible, however, because the owner frequently wanders from the patient at hand to all sorts of unrelated subjects.

"How's her appetite?" I might ask.

"Aw Doc, she eats corn and hay, what we've got of it. 'Course because of last summer's dry weather around here, I ain't got but a few bales of hay left. You know, it just don't rain right like it used to when I was growin' up. I believe it's on account of all that concrete they're pourin' in big cities and on them interstate highways. It's messin' up nature's order of things."

"Yes sir" is the only appropriate reply.

Second, once the history is taken, it is important to extend the conversation beyond veterinary matters. I believe a good veterinarian will show an interest in the client's family.

"How's Miss Emma Lou doing?" I might ask. "I heard she's been down with rheumatism lately."

"Aw Doc, you just don't know how she's suffered."

Miss Emma might not be a "Miss" at all. She might be the client's wife, or mother, or sister. But it's not uncommon in the South to refer to an older female member of the family as "Miss." Somehow it seems more respectful than calling her by her given name, yet less formal than saying "Mrs. Jones."

"Well, did Junior get hired on down at the sawmill?" I might say next.

"You bet, Doc. They say he's the best worker they've ever had down there. He's unloadin' logs right now, but they claim they're gonna move him on into the sawmill this summer."

"That's good! I knew the boy would make something out of himself."

Third, and equally important, is to pass compliments on the family dog, no matter how wormy, mangy, or ugly the canine may be. The farmer may even hate the dog, but no gesture carries as much public relations benefit as "bragging on" the dog, as a Southerner calls this activity. Any visitor who criticizes or abuses the family dog probably will not be invited back. In fact, violence could erupt toward the ill-tongued person.

As Mr. C. Y. and I walked toward the barn discussing the brilliance of his family cur, a hyena-bulldog hybrid-looking thing, the odor emanating from the barn increased in intensity. Finally, we stood before the stall and Mr. C. Y. commenced the task of unraveling the series of baling wire latches that secured the door.

I could hear an occasional shuffle and bumping sound from within the stall, which indicated to me that the patient was still ambulatory. That was good, since it is much easier to remove the placenta from a cow when both remover and removee are standing rather than being sprawled on the cold mucky ground.

After thirty seconds of fiddling with the wires, the door suddenly sprung open and there stood what surely must have been the ugliest cow in all of Alabama. The top of her back was streaked with long white hair, while the rest of her body was a bluish-gray color, occasionally ticked with faint white spots. She had long, mulelike ears and large goggle eyes which stared daggers at her intruders.

As she turned and pointed her rear parts in our direction, I could see a long slimy mass of putrid membranes dangling from her reproductive tract. The smell was stifling and was made even worse by the occasional air currents that swirled in underneath the stall and funneled out through the open door.

I quickly tossed the lariat over her head, made a temporary halter, and handed the loose end over to Mr. C. Y. He quickly looped the rope around the corner post and took up the slack. The cow offered only token resistance to the restraint, which indicated to me that she was feeling under the weather.

Soon I was scrubbing the cow's rear parts with well water and lye soap. It should be pointed out that nowhere in the medical textbooks or grand annals of bovine gynecology is the use of lye soap recommended. These books would recommend something more germicidal, foamy, and red in color. However, there are times when one uses what is at hand.

Lye soap is a homemade concoction made of lard or grease, lye, which is sodium hydroxide, and water. The mixture is contained in an iron pot, under which a fire has been built. The greasy mass must be constantly stirred with a long wooden paddle for several hours until the proper consistency is formed. Then the fire is allowed to go out and the soap is cooled naturally. By the next day it has taken on a firm consistency. It is cut into double-fist-size chunks and then stored in the smokehouse or storm cellar.

All this doesn't sound like much work, and actually it isn't, except that the stirring paddle is attended by a young boy who nearly barbecues himself over the flames. Also, the smoke constantly billows into his eyes and is being drawn into his sensitive nostrils. It is just one of many objectionable but necessary chores that had to be done by children back in older times.

If a lye soap user is not careful, the potent stuff will take off both hide and hair. So I was right careful to use sparing amounts as I soaped up the cow's rear end. After the second scrub, the area in question was squeaky clean and ready for a more detailed veterinary inspection.

However, as I turned to put on the clean shoulder-length glove, the cow decided at that moment to answer nature's call, which completely contaminated the squeaky-clean field that I had just prepared. This was not unexpected, since it is standard operating procedure for a cow to behave in such an uncooperative manner. I accomplished rescrub in short order and put on my glove.

Just as I inserted my lubricated and gloved arm elbow-deep into the innards of the cow, the barn door squeaked open and a large figure lumbered over to the stall.

"Where you been, Joe Bob? I thought you was gonna help hold this cow!" Mr. C. Y. said. "Here, grab aholt of this here rope."

Subsequent conversation revealed that Joe Bob was Mr. C. Y.'s son-in-law, a semiprofessional deer hunter, occasional pulpwood cutter, full-time good guy, and available veterinary assistant whenever cattle were being doctored or pigs castrated. He was just a big old boy, about six feet five and weighing nearly 275 pounds. Strong as a Tennessee mule, he could manhandle most any cow or bring a horse to its knees with the grip of his mighty fists.

According to Mr. C. Y., he had one fault. One morning several years before, he had "fell out," or fainted, in a muddy hog lot while assisting his well-known uncle, Carney Sam Jenkins, with some pig castrations. After that falling-out spell, Carney had dubbed him "Sinkin'" Jenkins and his numerous collapses after that were a constant source of hilarity, and concern, for the populace.

Some people refer to this fainting phenomenon as "white-eyeing." Sometimes just before a person goes into a faint, his eyes seem to rotate in their sockets, which reveals just the white portion of the eye. Therefore, a sudden rotation of eyeballs into the white should be considered an early warning for nearby observers.

Such a faint should not require a mad dash to the nearest phone with a request for the paramedics. Instead, cold water to the face or a couple of jaw-ringing slaps work very nicely in bringing the victim back to consciousness.

I immediately became concerned about Joe Bob since I was afraid that he might injure himself if he "fell out" while helping me restrain the present patient. But I continued working, keeping one eye on the potential fainter.

The rotten placenta was slowly dropping out, inch by inch, as my fingers carefully loosened its attachments inside the uterus. Meanwhile, Joe Bob was offering a commentary on deer-hunting techniques, the sorry state of government giveaway programs, and, most important, the status of Southeastern Conference football. I wondered how he could know so much about so many faraway subjects, since he said he didn't read much and didn't own a TV set. Suddenly the odor became obnoxiously intense and when the full mass of placenta dropped to the ground with a resounding "plop," Joe Bob suddenly stopped talking, cleared his throat, and gagged. Then his eyes rolled up in his head.

"Better grab that rope, Mr. C. Y.," I yelled, "Sinkin' is fixing to go down!"

I've noticed that no two people faint alike. In my observation, the most popular way to pass out is the stiff-legged fall over. They look like a standing board that is suddenly released from a firm grip. When they go down, they clear away everything in their path. Joe Bob, on the other hand, simply collapsed, dishrag fashion, into a heap on the ground. He fell atop neither cow nor man, broke no boards, nor did he make any unusual noises. The cow looked down at the crumpled mass of humanity at her hooves and sniffed it once before turning her head in the other direction. Obviously the still form did not meet with her approval.

"Don't worry about him, Doc, he'll come to in a minute," Mr. C. Y. said slowly. "Uh, I reckon I don't feel too pert myself." With that he too went over, in the classical stiff-legged manner. He keeled over fast, up against the feed trough, then ricocheted over against the chest wall of the cow before flopping directly onto the comatose Joe Bob. As before, the cow took one sniff at the carcass at her feet and looked away in disgust.

"Oh Lord! What a mess!" I mumbled to myself, my right arm now shoulder-deep, inserting sulfa urea boluses into the uterine horns of the cow. "Why can't I be like those big-time vets up North who never stain their spotless white coveralls, and have expert assistants who never pass out at the first sign of a disagreeable aroma?"

The bovine species is not known for high intelligence quotients. However, a cow is real smart about knowing when someone has quit holding the other end of her halter. It took my patient less than thirty seconds to figure out that since there were two prone bodies underneath her brisket, she was free. That's when even more fun started.

The cow started galloping clockwise around the stall periphery. I was sure that she needed the exercise, but because my right arm was still deep in her rear parts, I was getting a lot more of it than she was. Somehow my arm was positioned in such an angle that I could not extract it from her, and the fact that she was kicking like a young colt further complicated my dilemma.

Every third revolution or so she would reverse her field and try lapping the stall in counterclockwise fashion. This was difficult for me because it snapped me around, almost dislocating my elbow, before bashing me into the wall.

Meanwhile, the two fainters were being beaten around by cow feet, flying buckets, and one half-addled veterinarian. Awakened by all the hoopla, they were now shaking their heads, trying to focus their eyes, and attempting to stand. They were slipping and sliding on all the slick substances on the stall floor. Mostly, they were stumbling around trying to avoid all the flying deadly weapons.

Finally, the door flew open and like a gazelle, the cow evacuated the room. With a loud boot-out-of-the-mud slurping noise, my arm took leave of her interior. Out the front door of the barn the cow fled, never looking back, into the pasture where she joined her dozen or so colleagues. She had obviously had her fill of human interference that day.

Turning my attention back inside the barn, I saw Mr. C. Y. and Joe Bob stumbling out zombielike, coughing and gagging, in the hallway where the mule-drawn wagon was stored. They were picking up handfuls of straw and swiping tentatively at the manure, placenta, and mud that decorated their overalls.

I don't know why, but I've always had a problem of being overcome with laughter when folks become nauseated while I am working on one of their animals. So while Joe Bob and Mr. C. Y. were coughing, gagging, slobbering, slurring their words, and staring at each other in glassy-eyed discomfort, I was trying hard not to give in to the fit of guffawing that was threatening to erupt from my jerking chest.

I grabbed a bucket and fled to the well, giggling while I ran and giggling when I lowered the empty bucket down into the water. By the time I returned to the fainters I had regained most of my composure and was offering them wet towels. They sheepishly accepted and made several swipes at their faces while shaking their heads and mumbling their apologies.

To ask if they needed medical attention or other help would have been inappropriate. They had already been humiliated enough, and any further embarrassment in front of a nonnative would be damaging to their pride. Even though it was a common occurrence, most figured that passing out or getting "stomach queasy" was a sign of weakness. Wives and girlfriends were not informed about such wimplike behavior for fear of retribution at some later date.

As I left the farm that day, I thought about the fainting phenomenon and just what caused the problem in some people, while others remained forever faint-free. Since I had never observed a single fainting spell in a female who was assisting me with an unpleasant and smelly task, I concluded that the affliction must be a defect somewhere in or on the male gene. Also, large men seem to be more prone to collapse than small men, and those who engage in rough-and-tough activities, such as athletics, are prime candidates. Many of these are troubled by offensive smells and the sight of blood.

I can still recall my first client-collapsing episode. It was a hot Saturday afternoon during my internship when a very pregnant lady and her huge, defensive-tackle-looking husband named Sampson brought their middle-aged cocker spaniel into the clinic for treatment of a severe and odoriferous ear infection, commonly known as "canker ear."

The lady was no more than five feet tall and weighed no more than a hundred pounds. Her man was in the vicinity of six feet six, weighed about two-fifty, and had only about two percent fat on his massive frame. He was, as the kennel boy said, "a hoss."

I was real concerned about the lady. She was sweating profusely as she waddled down the hall ahead of the big guy, and the thought went through my mind that she might just go into labor there at the clinic.

The thought made me sweat, too. She wanted to pick up "Poochie" and put him on the table, but I insisted on doing it myself. Sampson didn't offer to help, but just stood there twitching his head, neck, and right shoulder like he was punch drunk.

As I cleaned out Poochie's smelly ears with cotton and alcohol, I heard a barely audible groan emerge from the man's throat. I looked over at him just in time to see drops of sweat big as hookworm pills rolling off his forehead and his eyes roll around backward in their sockets.

"What is it, honey?" the soon-to-be-mom exclaimed. "Dear, you look so peaked and—"

She couldn't finish the sentence because Sampson had started to fall to the checkered linoleum of the clinic floor.

His legs stiffened and his hands blindly clawed for the table as he listed seriously to the right. His wife patted on his upper arm lovingly, but had the good sense to move outside of the probable path of his collapse. Since I was on the opposite side of the table from him, I left the shaking dog alone on the table and tried to get around to help block Sampson's fall. However, by the time I got there, he had already crashed to the floor like a huge, branchy pine tree. His fingernails made horrible skin-crawling noises as they scraped the metal table. Then his shoulder caught the edge of a tray of instruments on a small stand at the end of the table and sent them scattering all over the floor. His head went crashing into the side of the old refrigerator, causing the door to fly open and spill rabies vaccine over the mass of instruments on the floor.

When his body met linoleum, it bounced a couple of times and the old building literally shook and rattled like an earthquake had hit. Then, for a brief instant, there was silence, except for vials of vaccine rolling around and bumping up against the wall.

Immediately the pregnant woman went into action. As I put a sofa cushion under her unconscious husband's head, she went to the sink, brought wet towels, and started applying the cool water to his face. The dog looked down, with head tilted in wonder, at the three individuals on the floor.

After a couple of minutes of cool water applications to his forehead and a couple of slaps to the face from his wife, the sleeping giant started to blink his eyes and rake instruments around with his hands.

Eventually, Sampson arose weakly and staggered out to his car with support from his faithful wife. Presently she returned and helped me finish with Poochie's ears.

"Aw, he's bad to faint," she said. "He even passed out during our wedding ceremony. I wonder what he'll do when the baby comes."

I heard later that he did have some light-headed moments in the OB ward. He never came into the clinic again, even though his wife brought the dog in many times after that. I reckon he was just too embarrassed to show his face there again.

It's obvious there are a lot of people out there who can't stand the sight of blood and are physically incapacitated when they catch a sniff or two of irregular odors. Those of us who work around these people should watch out for them and be sure they don't hurt themselves when they collapse. Or with large people like Sinkin' Jenkins and Sampson, be sure they don't hurt *us*. I just stay out of their "fall line."

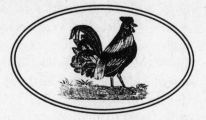

Chapter 14

WINTERTIME IN SOUTHWEST Alabama is not particularly difficult compared to Northern winters. Most days in December and January are pleasant enough, although it is not uncommon to see the temperature drop into the low twenties. Occasionally, it reaches the teens, but rarely does it fall into the single digits. Single-digit weather is called "bad cold." Occasional snow, or even the threat of a few flakes, calls for early school and shirt factory dismissals, since even a half inch of the white stuff results in chaos on the roadways. Of course it does not delay more important pursuits, such as deer hunting or veterinary calls.

But the thing that makes wintertime miserable is the cold, thirty-five- to forty-degree rain. Even if it's not raining, thirty-five-degree weather with high humidity seems to penetrate to the bone of both man and beast. Man can dress in layers of clothing and peel off a layer or two as the temperature rises, but cattle are not afforded that luxury. Another problem arises for veterinarians working with bovine obstetrics. It is very difficult to deliver a calf, perform a cesarian section, or replace a large prolapsed uterus while wearing several layers of shirts and coats. Stripping down to bare chest or tee shirt gives one much more arm strength and flexibility but it also increases the chance of frostbite. Then again, it also increases the speed with which the procedure is performed!

After driving our station wagon over wintertime Choctaw County roads and pastures, it became apparent that its low chassis was not appropriate for such use. I had already knocked off the muffler, scraped the rear end going over rough railroad crossings, hung the bumper on a pine stump, and acquired dents in several spots from unruly cows and colicky mules. Flat tires were a common occurrence.

In addition, the interior had developed a peculiar odor, normal to me, but perhaps a little offensive to others who might have been riding in the car, such as a load of kids going to a birthday party. It was not only the odor of mule leg liniment, dog dips, and boar hog vitamins; I was calling on more swine farms than I had anticipated, and that odor had permeated the fabric of the seats and floor mats. Jan and I both laughed about the smell and said it had the aroma of money, and for that we were grateful. However, even a veterinarian doesn't want to go to church or the PTA reeking of essence of pigsty.

Since I was out in the country a large portion of every day, Jan had no transportation in case of an emergency. Of course, we had new friends we could call upon if necessary, but I was growing more and more concerned about my family having to depend upon others for help.

Then there was the fact that all my large animal clients drove pickup trucks and many of them had made jokes about my ground-scraping station wagon and how it wasn't going to last very long the way I was driving it into pastures and hog lots. There was no overt pressure exerted on me to buy a truck, but it was a little embarrassing to drive up to the stockyard or a cattlemen's meeting behind the wheel of a station wagon and park it in amongst a hundred trucks. It just didn't feel right.

It was odd how pickup trucks were becoming more and more comfortable and luxurious. It hadn't been but a few years since a truck was little more than a bare, chromeless, depressing item of machinery hanging around behind the barn. It was a useful apparatus all right, but only for taking a few bales of hay to the cows, delivering a load of cantaloupes up to the farmer's market, or hauling a couple of bluetick hounds over to Grandpaw's for a nocturnal coon hunt.

The first one I ever drove belonged to my uncle Frank. It was hard to crank and the springs in the seat tortured your behind. It shimmied and it knocked; it was good for hauling barley. But there was no gusto involved in driving it, nor was the experience worthy of the bragging of even a sixteen-year-old.

Nowadays, pickup trucks are much more comfortable vehicles that make life easier for folks like farmers and veterinarians. One noted

dirt-road psychologist has said that the benefits of pickup truck ownership extend far beyond the obvious physical benefits of the ability to
haul various materials.

It has been noted that truck drivers are happier, feel better about
themselves, and are able to tolerate the pressures of everyday life in
better fashion than drivers of sedans. Truck drivers arrive at work in a
better frame of mind, and once they are in the workplace, seem more
immune to the harassment of the one or two idiots that seem to plague
every job site or office.

This feeling of confidence and well-being may be due to the way the
good radio music tends to permeate the warmth of a truck cab. Somehow music just sounds better in a truck. The driver drifts into a mel-
low and mesmerized mood, which tends to persist for hours. Another
theory is that the euphoric feeling comes about simply because the
truck driver knows deep down in his heart that he's doing right. I've
never heard Scripture quoted that refers to the goodness of pickup
driving, but I wouldn't be surprised if there's not an obscure passage
somewhere in the Good Book along that line.

Also, since the occupants of a pickup truck are higher off the road
than those seated in sedans, it gives them the advantage of being able
to see things along the road that others cannot. They can see over the
bushes and beyond into the fields, pastures, and woods and enjoy
interesting sights there, and they can look down at the sedan owners
creeping along the ground below.

As wonderful as truck ownership is, it has a couple of minor disad-
vantages. It will seat the typical four-member family, although somewhat intimately. However, if you plan to take eight head of kin out for
barbecue when it's raining or snowing, you do have a problem.

Another problem that surfaces is that covetous non–truck owners
frequently want to borrow their neighbor's pickup. These people have
the gall to expect to haul things such as manure, rocks, tree limbs,
scrap iron, and other scratch-prone items in the back of someone's
truck! The astute owner must tactfully refer all such requests to the
local U-Haul headquarters.

In spite of all these problems and possible entanglements, I still
wanted that truck. In fact, I knew that I had contracted a serious case
of the Truck Buying Fever.

I have observed many cases of the TB Fever over the years in my friends, family, and clients. The condition is characterized by depression, long stares at almost any truck that passes within sight, and ink-stained fingers from constantly fingering through the "trucks for sale" ads in the newspaper. Sufferers also slow down while driving by used vehicle lots or parked trucks with signs in their windows, and make quick late-night and Sunday excursions to the Chevrolet and Ford dealerships. I had the disease and I knew the only cure was to buy one. I also knew that the only kind I could afford would be a "previously owned" one, perhaps two or three years old.

It's incredible how a good truck salesman can sniff out and diagnose even the most obscure case of Truck Buying Fever in his territory. It may be that he can smell it, or perhaps he keeps a close eye on the street, watching for those who go by his lot real slow with their necks craned. Perhaps he has spies watching for these fevered individuals. Somehow, the world's best truck salesman found me.

"Dr. McCormack, I have a dog that needs to be vaccinated against distemper and rabies, and he needs deworming," the man said on the phone. "When could you get to it?"

"How about late tomorrow?" I suggested.

"Great, I'll be over after work," he declared.

"OK. Who is this, please?"

"My name is Clatis Tew. We haven't met, but you have treated several of my neighbors' pets and you've visited some farms in the south end of the county owned by my friends and customers."

Clatis Tew! What a great-sounding name. I've always enjoyed hearing a person's name for the first time and trying to figure out what kind of work he or she does. When I first heard Mr. Tew's name, I knew he was a master salesman of some kind. I had to inquire about his vocation.

"Do you work at the paper mill?" I asked.

"No, I'm a sales representative for McPhearson Chevrolet," he replied with enthusiasm.

I knew it! I just knew it! Somehow he had learned of my truck need and wasted no time in contacting me in the cleverest possible way. He was bringing me a little business, figuring that he would spend twenty dollars or so, but I would spend hundreds in return. He would probably even come over to the house in the very truck he intended to sell me, with it all washed up and shiny, his fine dog riding proudly in the back. I prepared to put up at least a token amount of sales resistance.

I've always thought it was important to develop a strong sales-resistance mechanism, especially in the South, in order to prevent bankruptcy. There is always a plethora of aluminum siding salesmen, burial plot pushers, fly-by-night roof painters whose watered-down application lasts only through the next rainstorm, and expert insurance agents who always convince you that you'll be graveyard dead in just hours, leaving your poor spouse penniless, in spite of what you thought would be a generous payoff benefit from your previous policy.

There are many good things out there to buy, thanks to good old American ingenuity, but you can't succumb to all your purchasing desires. Boiled peanuts, Moon Pies, Goo Goo bars, and barbecue sandwiches are all necessities of good Southern living, but without some personal restraint, such items will nickel, dime, and dollar you straight to the poorhouse, to say nothing of more expensive items.

Right at dusk the next afternoon, there came a sharp rap on the front door.

"Hello, I'm Clatis Tew!" said the man, sticking out his hand. "I've brought my little dog for his vaccinations."

"Good, good." I replied. "Where is he?"

"Out in the truck. I didn't know whether to bring him in or not."

When I stepped out onto the porch, I spied the truck. Just as I had predicted, the mixed-breed dog was standing in the back, with his paws up on the side of the body. The Chevy was a short-bed type, a 1961 or 1962 model, mud tires on the rear, and a dark blue so shiny that it hurt my eyes. It had obviously been washed and waxed by the best man they had in the service department. The baited hook was dangling right in front of my eyes and I seemed to be losing control. I felt my sales resistance oozing away. At that moment I realized that I was suffering from a chronic case of pickup truck addiction.

"Clatis, bring your dog around to the carport. I've made a little exam room out of the storage room."

My initial practice plan had been to deal primarily with large animals, making trips to the farms in the area as called. It quickly became apparent, however, that there was a huge demand for small-animal veterinary medicine. At first, I provided house call service for pets, but it was less time-consuming for them to come to me since I would frequently be in the country all day. I tried to see the dogs and cats in the late afternoon or night after everyone's workday was over.

Although it was inadequate for its purpose, we had fixed up the small storage area at the end of the carport with a table, shelves for drugs, and a couple of temporary cages where I could keep pets overnight after surgery. That was the best I could do until I could see whether the populace would support an animal clinic. The way things had been going, I believed they would, so Jan and I had been looking around town for a suitable place to rent or a lot to purchase. I had long ago come up with a clinic floor plan that I liked and that wouldn't cost an arm and leg. All I needed was a little more time and a lot more money.

As Clatis and I examined, vaccinated, and dewormed his dog, we visited. Even though he had been brought up in the county to the south, he amazed me with his knowledge of Choctaw County. Clatis repeated much information Carney Sam had already told me about the history of the county, politics, and in what direction the leaders thought the county was going.

Soon we were walking toward the gleaming truck and depositing the dog in the back.

"Dr. John, whenever you're ready to get yourself a truck, I hope you'll keep me in mind," he said, handing me a card. "I don't know if you've seen all of our county roads yet, but your business is going to require something more rugged than a nice station wagon." He looked over at the muddy wagon and shook his head back and forth.

"John, you're gonna ruin your wife's car if you're not careful," he said.

"Well, I don't know if I can afford to buy a truck right now . . . " I replied.

"John, you can't afford not to!" he exclaimed. "Now just take this little Chevy right here. It might just be the ticket for your line of work. It's just two years old and was owned by an elderly gentleman who only drove it to church twice every week, and to the doctor and to get groceries once a month. It's hardly broken in!"

Now he was on a roll, slapping the hood, kicking a tire, slamming a door, and wiping at a tiny speck of dirt on the rear fender with his handkerchief. He opened the hood and we peered down into the classic in-line six-cylinder engine that looked like it had received recent tender loving care.

The interior was spotless and still had the new smell to it. The odometer indicated there had been some 26,000 miles driven, and the cigarette lighter had never been used. A quick peek in the back revealed not even a single scratch.

"How much do you want for it?" I inquired, after taking a gander up underneath.

"I don't know exactly. Didn't bring my book with me, so I'd have to check back at the office."

"Uh huh."

"Tell you what let's do," he exclaimed. "Let's drive uptown and I'll get all the papers and we'll see what we can come up with. Here, you drive." I'm sure that's part of their basic training in sales school. Before you quote a price, make sure the prospect gets behind the wheel. By that time most buyers have the hook, line, and sinker in their mouths and they are nibbling around on the bait.

It drove as good as it looked. It negotiated the big hole in the road with comfort, then climbed the hill into town with ease. By the time I pulled up in front of the dealership, the hook was solidly set. Clatis went inside, while I continued my inspection of things I had forgotten earlier. I fingered the inside of the exhaust pipe and found it was dry. I checked the shock absorbers, looked at the spare tire, examined the master cylinder, the radiator, the windshield wipers, and the lights. The only problem I could find was the rear bumper. Apparently, the previous owner had hung a pine stump or cemetery marker on the edge of the right portion of the bumper and had sprung it slightly. It pointed upward at a forty-five-degree angle and slightly outward.

As I continued my inspection, I could see what was happening inside the building through the huge plate glass windows. Clatis was rummaging through a small box inside one of those little partitioned rooms where car deals are negotiated. Then he went into another see-through room and put his head close to someone else's, probably that of the "head" man.

While I was under the truck checking for oil and muffler leaks, I heard Clatis, then saw his shoes as he neared the truck.

"Find anything wrong under there, Doc?" he questioned.

"Nope, not a thing yet," I replied, as I slid out and stood up. "Except that bumper."

"Doc, I'm not gonna let you drive something off this lot that's not right. You're gonna be in this town a long time and I'm gonna be here a long time too. Now how do you think I'd feel, waving at you on the road every day if I let you have a vehicle that won't do."

As predicted, I drove the truck home, because they couldn't locate "the papers." I believe this is the final lesson and lecture at car-selling school. If you are sure of your product, let the potential customer take it home for the night or for the weekend. The vehicle will sell itself.

A couple of days later we signed the papers and I owned my first truck. This purchase of a used pickup truck, perhaps minor to many, was a major step for me. It provided dependable dirt-road transportation, freed up the car for Jan and the kids, and made some of my clients take me a little more seriously.

I believe the purchase of this truck taught me a lesson valuable to anyone going into business, especially in a small town. You can't sell a service or a product that "won't do" to somebody you'll be waving to on the road every day. Clatis was right, and I have never forgotten it.

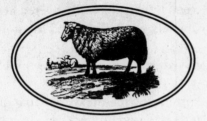

Chapter 15

MY NEW TRUCK gave me a new sense of freedom. I found myself plunging down logging roads and challenging briar-infested pastures on a routine basis without fear of damage. I knew that if I mired up in the mud, the farmer could tractor me out and my truck would usually be none the worse. I wondered how I had ever done without it.

I also discovered the necessity of always carrying a shovel around in the truck. Some farmers, when they spied my shovel, would make smart aleck remarks, saying that it was there primarily for digging the graves of expired cows. Those were the same farmers who claimed that buzzards constantly followed my truck, so they could easily locate their next banquet. I just laughed along with them, since they seemed to enjoy such joshing so much. But one thing I knew for sure: in the presence of substantial amounts of both road and off-road mud, it was written in stone that I would eventually get stuck in it.

Not long after I got my truck, Miss Ruby McCord, proprietor of McCord's General Store and Service Station, called late one cold and blustery night right before Christmas. Apparently some coon hunters had found one of her cows in labor. From her description over the phone, it was apparent that it was a breech birth.

Miss Ruby was always proper and correct in her conversation. She didn't use any slang or regular cowboy jargon when describing day-to-day activities. She would never refer to the male cow as a "bull," for instance, because the word "bull" was too coarse for sensitive ears. Instead, she referred to the bull as "the Sunday cow." I often heard my grandmother use the same careful phraseology.

"Doctor, one of my brood cows is encountering some serious difficulty. Some local raccoon hunters have discovered her over near an old cotton house approximately one mile behind my store," she said, carefully selecting her words.

"Yes, I understand. Can you tell me what the problem is?" I figured it must be a labor case.

"Yes, of course. Apparently, she is experiencing difficulty in giving birth, and from what the raccoon hunters have related to me, I suspect that she has a breech presentation, because there is evidence of a fetal tail protruding from the cow's rear parts." It must have been a strain for Miss Ruby to describe a medical problem that involved a cow's rear parts. I could almost see her red face and shuffling feet as she talked into the old wall-mounted telephone out in the unheated hallway of her hundred-year-old home.

For a normal delivery to take place, the bovine fetus must be presented front feet first, followed by the nose lying at the level of the carpus, commonly called the knees of the front limbs. Any other presentation is abnormal, although a fetus may be born without difficulty if it comes backward. But it is almost impossible if it is breeched.

A breech presentation means that the fetus tries to come "butt" first but the rear legs are retained. Not only are they retained, but they are way forward, almost out of reach of even the longest of veterinary arms. Experienced and observant cow owners often recognize the problem because the patient has been in labor for quite some time, gradually becoming exhausted and finally involuntarily terminating the normal birthing process. They may also observe a portion of fetal tail protruding from the birth canal. Inexperienced persons eventually realize there is a problem, but they often don't see that telltale tail.

"The raccoon hunters indicated that they will be waiting for you at the gate and will escort you to the cow. I regret I am indisposed and cannot accompany you to the pasture."

At least there would be someone there to help. One problem that I constantly seemed to have was making farm calls to assist elderly gentlemen or widows who were unable to help with their cows. This was understandable, and I found that sometimes I could actually get the job done faster when there weren't people there trying to help where they were liable to get hurt.

When I reached the gate on the dirt road behind Miss Ruby's store, there were three hunters standing out in the road waving lights and

lanterns. They were attired in the latest hunter's garb and had big
knives strapped to their sides. Each had some type of powerful light
attached to his cap, in addition to a hand-carried light.

When I slid to a stop in front of the gate, the hunters all rushed to
my open window, each trying to talk and be the first to tell the vet
what was happening and where the bovine patient was located.

It quickly became apparent that the three hunters were engaging in
an activity common on many night hunts. I knew from their rank
smell, their slurry speech, and their unsteady gaits that they had enthusiastically been consuming alcoholic substances. No sooner had I realized this than one retrieved a bottle from the vast game pocket of his
hunting vest.

"How 'bout a drank?" he slurred, shakily extending the bottle
toward the windshield. In the dim lantern light, I noticed the liquid in
the labeled bottle appeared dark-colored, so I assumed it was "red"
whiskey, so called because it had been legally made and store bought.

Immediately another hunter produced a quart fruit jar which was
about a third full of a clear liquid. I assumed this was "white" whiskey,
or genuine, homemade Choctaw County moonshine liquor.

"Uh, no thanks," I replied. "I better see about Miss Ruby's cow. Can
y'all come show me where the cow is?" I asked.

Soon the three hunters were squeezed in the cab alongside me and
all the veterinary paraphernalia that I was hauling.

"Which way is the cow?" I asked.

"Bear to the right, she's down this hill in that pine thicket," one
advised.

"Sho is a nice truck you got, Doc. It smells brand new," said Tyrone,
one of the hunters.

I was impressed that Tyrone's olfactory system could detect new-
ness in the pickup's atmosphere. To me, it was smelling more like
moonshine breath and old sweat. I wondered how long I could take it
before bailing out for fresh air. I eased the truck down the suddenly
muddy hill, rolling down the window with one hand and wrestling
the steering wheel with the other.

"Yonder she is, lying under that pine sapling," announced the one
mashed up against the passenger-side door. "Doc, you can drive right
up to 'er and lay your rope right on 'er!"

"Sure," I thought to myself. "Just walk up to her, rub her nose, and say hello, then simply put a halter on her head and go on about your business!"

No cow in labor, unless she is stupefied, paralyzed, or disabled, can resist the urge to stand when a stranger, especially one with veterinary intentions, approaches. She may have been reposing in the same spot since sunup, and paid no heed to the farmer or hired man, but when the veterinarian arrives, she can be expected to spring to her feet and sprint like a scatback toward the most remote corner of the property.

"Y'all stay right here in the truck now and don't get out until I call you, OK?" I said quietly, as I drove up so the cow would be blinded by the left headlight. Then I eased the door open and slipped all the way around the truck, with lariat in hand, stopping close to the right fender.

The ability to throw a rope with some degree of accuracy was important at that time. Important, that is, if the vet had any intention of restraining the cow and taking care of the problem for which he was summoned. Corrals were scarce and getting the patient to the barn or an enclosure on short notice was often nigh impossible.

The first thing a cow roper does, even before tossing the loop, is locate something substantial to which the free end of the rope can be tied immediately after the cow is caught. Otherwise, the roper may find himself being dragged through the woods by a panicked bovine whose rate of speed is remarkable, considering that she is also burdened with an eighty-pound fetus and an udder the size of a yearling turkey. I picked out a small tree nearby.

Then I twirled the rope over my head, and let it fly, just as the cow noticed my movement. Luckily, the loop fell cleanly over her large horns and head as she stood and commenced her great skedaddle to the woods.

"Now! Help me! Come on!" I screamed, as the cow started taking up slack in the thirty feet of rope while I frantically tried in vain to pass it around the small tree. Suddenly bodies appeared and I could see multiple arms reaching for the rope, which was now wiggling through the grass and bushes. Amid a lot of whooping and hollering, Tyrone, the most athletic but dumbest of the hunters, dove upon the rope and was quickly dragged into the bushy night. From the darkness, I could hear the popping of twigs and the snapping of branches, accompanied by the sound of hunting pants sliding through briars and an occasional loud human grunt.

Before long I detected the loud, raspy breathing of the cow, which indicated she was beginning to choke down from the rope that was encircling her neck. It also meant she had probably tired of dragging Tyrone's two-hundred-pound body through the underbrush.

"Tyrone's got 'er, Doc! He's got 'er! Come on!" a voice yelled from down in the trees, some fifty yards away. I quickly grabbed my flashlight, bucket, jug of water, disinfectant soap, calf jack, and black bag, and half ran, half stumbled down the miniravine to where the commotion was continuing. It seemed the cow objected to the way she was being pulled and pushed toward the tree of choice, so a fracas had developed between her and the coon hunters, complete with bellowing, yelling, kicking, and the wild waving of arms. Finally, she was pulled up close to the tree and the rope tied.

"Thanks a lot, guys," I said. That's when I noticed Tyrone. His clothes were torn, his cap gone, his face scratched, and briars were protruding from various points of his clothing.

"Are you OK, Tyrone?"

"Yeah, why?" he replied.

It is impossible to avoid bruises and knots after being dragged fifty yards over stumps, brush, and briars. I figured he had been preanesthetized. I had noticed on previous occasions that when individuals partook of strong drink, especially the potent Choctaw County variety, their responses to painful stimuli were greatly reduced.

As I washed up the cow's rear parts for my examination, I heard the baying of a hound some half mile to the east.

"Listen! Listen!" whispered one hunter, the one whose ears were still functioning. Quiet ensued for several seconds.

"That's ole Preacher, and he's got a coon treed in that patch of woods by the railroad. We gotta go to 'im!"

"You sure that's Preacher? Sounds more like old Lou to me," Tyrone allowed. At that point Tyrone probably couldn't have detected the difference between the barks of Preacher, old Lou, or a laughing hyena.

"Can y'all wait just a few minutes? I might need some help jacking this calf out of this cow," I said.

A calf jack, also called a calf puller, or fetal extractor, consists of a winch, handle, and cable device attached to one end of a six- to eight-foot rod. On the opposite end of the rod is a Y-shaped piece which is placed against the hind legs of the laboring cow. The cable is then attached to an obstetrical chain or strap which has just been secured to the protruding legs of the fetus. The fetus is then slowly extracted, matching the cow's pushing and straining efforts. A fetal extractor is a useful piece of equipment when used correctly and with judgment. If not used properly, it can injure the fetus and paralyze the cow.

Ideally, there should be two people working with a calf jack. One should work the winch and the other should attend the birth canal area and the fetus, to be sure everything is proceeding as planned.

By then my right arm had entered the birth canal and detected a deceased fetus, so decomposed that when I removed my hand, a horribly foul odor filled the air. I knew then that I would soon be working alone.

"Man! Somethin' stinks!" yelled the one holding the head rope. Obviously, he was downwind.

"Here Tyrone, hold this rope, quick!" Then he staggered up against a large tree while making coughing, gagging, and groaning noises.

Several feet behind the cow, hunter number two moaned and said something about not feeling too good either, then he started running away and retching. I quickly looked at Tyrone and discovered that his mouth was half open, his tongue making in-and-out movements. He was salivating profusely.

"Y'all hurry back," I yelled, "Tyrone's next!"

Then I got tickled as usual. I wish there were some way I could control myself in this type of situation, but I have given it up as a lost cause. I tried to stifle myself while hiding behind the cow, who by then had accepted her fate and was cooperating better than I had anticipated.

In minutes they were all back, wearing sheepish grins.

"Doc, how can you stand that smell?" one asked. "Don't it make you sick at your stomach?"

"What smell? I don't smell anything," I declared solemnly, while pulling and tugging on a fetal leg until it was up in normal position. It also brought out more odor.

"Doc, I hate to leave, but we gotta go. Preacher's treed over yonder, and I got to be at work at midnight," one said from the darkness.

"I understand, and I really do appreciate your help. Maybe someday I can return the favor," I said.

Then they were off, walking in the direction of the far-off barking dog. I could hear them discussing the robustness of the bad smell until their voices trailed off to an occasional murmur.

Freed of regurgitating assistants and my own giggle apparatus, I soon had both rear legs of the fetus up and protruding from the birth canal. Then I pumped a half gallon of lubricant onto the rear end of the fetus before beginning the actual delivery with the calf jack.

After much jacking, twisting, and vocal urging, the lifeless fetus popped out and flopped onto the pine straw. As expected, the cow went down midway through the procedure, which made the whole process more tedious. It is difficult to work a calf jack when the patient is sitting cow fashion.

I quickly made a manual examination of the reproductive tract, introduced some sulfa boluses, injected penicillin, and released the neck rope. A slap on her rump produced instant results, and the cow hastily fled through the night, never looking back at her deceased offspring. I could see why she wanted no part of the thing that had caused her so much annoyance, but I have never understood how a cow can stand so quickly after a major operation and immediately run like the wind, as if nothing has happened.

There was only enough water to wash a portion of the stinking gunk off my hands and arms, so I put my equipment back in the truck to clean later. I knew I must have had a horrible odor, but I could smell nothing. My olfactory system had adapted to it in the past thirty minutes.

The truck cranked right up, much to my delight. One of a large animal veterinarian's greatest pleasures is a truck that starts after its headlights have been shining over a late-night patient for a long time.

In order to make my way out of the woods pasture, I had the option of backing the vehicle up the hill or going down the hill for fifty yards or so, making a right turn, then coming back up by the fence where the terrain was more level. I chose to go down the hill.

All went well as I eased down by the edge of the pine thicket and out into the knee-high sage grass pasture. Just as I proceeded into the grass, I thought I spied a wet spot, so I goosed the accelerator slightly to get on through it quickly. Unfortunately, it was a *very* wet spot, apparently fed by a series of wet weather springs.

The truck hit bottom, right up to the axle. I felt the cold chill of panic ascend up my spinal cord. I was in a passel of trouble, cold, dog tired, smelly, and miles from the nearest help. After briefly trying to escape from my predicament, I found that the rear wheels were turning in the holes they had made, but the rear axle that was snug to the ground was the problem.

Fuming, fussing, and feeling sorry for myself, I abandoned the truck and started the long walk to a telephone. I knew that Miss Ruby had a phone and I also knew that her house was approximately a mile away across the swamp as the crow flies. But I was afraid of getting lost in that swamp and never being seen again. So I decided to go the long way around, which meant that I had a mile to walk down the gravel road to the store, then another mile back up the paved road to her house.

When people are cold, stinking, hungry, and mad at the world, they usually question their choice of vocations. As I tromped and kicked clods, I wondered and complained out loud.

"Why is it that everybody in Choctaw County waits until it's black dark to call the veterinarian? Why don't I just sleep all day and work all night, just like the night man down at the filling station?

"Maybe someday I'll sell out this practice and become a learned professor in a veterinary school somewhere," I mumbled. "Then I'd have an easy job, always flying all over the country giving talks and fiddling around doing research on some obscure, meaningless disease."

But I decided that wouldn't work for me, because it would be difficult to answer the questions of the highly intelligent students.

Not a single car came along during the entire walk, but a bread truck going the opposite direction nearly blew me off the road as I approached Miss Ruby's house.

I remembered that she had a yard full of dogs, many of which were mean weimaraners. When I approached the front gate, the racket commenced. After a leadoff bark or two, there was an explosion of barking and snarling dogs, running back and forth along the fence line and jumping up and down as if on springs. It sounded as if there were four or five of them.

"Miss Rubbbyyy!" I yelled. "Hello, Miss Rubbbyyy!"

When the dogs heard me calling Miss Ruby's name, they went into an absolute fit of trumpeting, as if some basic brain response had been stimulated.

"*Miss Rubbbyyy!* Are you awake? This is Dr. McCormack! I need to use your phone!"

The canine cacophony continued for five minutes or so, and just as I was trying to decide what my next move should be, a light came on in the big hallway. Through the window I could see a figure moving slowly toward the front door.

"*Who is it? What do you want?*" she yelled, although somewhat less loudly than the dogs.

"Miss Ruby, this is Dr. McCormack. Your cow is fine, but now my truck is stuck over in the pasture. Will you call Jan and ask her to come get me?" Certainly she would know how to get to Miss Ruby's house since we had recently been there to vaccinate her dogs against rabies.

"*Who?* Who is it?" she reyelled. The dogs continued their hulla-baloo practice. I desperately wanted to bend over, pick up a large handful of prune-size rocks, and rain them down spitefully on the pack of disorderly beasts. I was cold, hungry, mad, sleepy, and was surely going to lose money on that farm call before it was all over.

"*THE COW DOCTOR!*" I screamed. "*My truck's broken down over yonder in your field.*" Surely the dogs would soon be hoarse and voice-less before I was, I hoped.

"*Buck Who?*" she retorted.

Now I was seething! My temper had just about reached the boiling point, not at Miss Ruby, but at the fool dogs, and at myself.

In a flash, I reached down and picked up a handful of the prunelike rocks, and in one quick motion, whistled them some thirty yards toward the head barker. One must have caught him in a vital spot because a split second after the thud, he let out a quick yelp and bee-lined it up under the front porch. Then there was a blessed silence, except for the ringing in my ears and an occasional growl. I closed my eyes and offered up a quick prayer, asking to be forgiven. I lowered my voice to a semiyell.

"Miss Ruby, it's Dr. John!"

"What's wrong, Doctuh?" It's amazing what you can get accom-plished without lots of barking and noise. Now she was out on the front porch and I was through the gate, striding up the walkway.

"I'm sorry, I didn't realize it was you. Sometimes I have to throw corncobs at these dogs to quieten them down," she said as I went up

the steps. "They're real good watchdogs, but sometimes they don't
know when to cease their barking. I suspect that some young ruffians
have been coming by here and throwing stones at them. That's what
makes them so nervous."

"Yes ma'am," I replied, with lips pursed and head lowered. I could
just envision this elderly lady throwing a corncob! I stopped about
halfway up the steps because of the smell.

"What about my cow?"

"Oh, she's fine. I corrected her problem but the calf was deceased.
She had been in labor too long." I didn't go into much detail because all
the gory details would have embarrassed us both. Words such as "pregnant," "afterbirth," "rotten fetus," and any reference to the places
where my arms had been working an hour ago were definitely taboo,
so I deleted those areas from my report.

"Doctuh, your clothes are terribly soiled and the aroma you present
is considerably less than fragrant," she pronounced. What a delight-
fully diplomatic way to inform someone that they stunk. I vowed to
remember her words.

"Well, your cow gave it to me after I worked with her for an
extended period."

"Oh, really! Then it's no wonder the raccoon hunters were so
explicit in their description of her condition," she exclaimed.

I wanted to tell her that the coon hunters presented an odor at least
as objectionable as the bovine patient. I wanted to tell her the cow
would probably have become nauseated at the stench of all that rotgut
whiskey if she had not possessed four stomachs of such cast-iron stur-
diness.

"Will you do me a favor please ma'am? Please call my wife and ask
her to come pick me up. My truck is mired up in the pasture and I'm
just too tired to fool with it tonight. I'll come back in the morning and
get it out."

"Of course. I'm sorry about your conveyance. Perhaps you could
enlist the aid of Mr. Jack Means, who has a John Deere tractor. He
lives about a mile south of my store and I'm sure you've visited his
farm on occasion."

"Yes ma'am. I might do that."

Then she disappeared back into the hall and I could see her dialing
the phone while reading my number off the back of the directory.

While she was phoning, I looked around to see what the dogs were up to. When one growled from under the porch, I drew back my arm as if to throw something and he yelped and scurried back under the house, bumping floor joists in his haste. Miss Ruby was probably right in thinking someone had been tormenting those dogs.

"*Hello,* is this Mrs. *McCormack?*" I heard her say. "Well, this is *Ruby McCord* just north of *Lisman, Alabama.*" She was yelling out some of the key words, while using a normal voice on others.

"The *Doctuh* asked me to . . ." then there was a short pause.

"Oh yes, *he's* alright, but he got his *conveyance mired up* and wants *you* to come *get* him." Then another pause, this time a little longer.

"*Yes, yes, I'll tell him.* Yes, all right. *Goodbye,* goodbye!"

It was normal telephone operating procedure to yell, or at least talk loud, when conversing over the phone at that time. I suppose it was because people figured since they were trying to talk to somebody a long way off, it was necessary to speak that way. Some of my kin say that I still yell over the phone; old habits die hard.

"She said she'd be here as quickly as possible, but it would take a few minutes to get the kids out of bed and bundled up. She seems like such a nice lady."

"She sure is. She takes real good care of those kids and me, plus handling the phone and taking care of the books."

"Well, it shouldn't take but about ten minutes or so. Would you like to come in out of the cold?" she asked, while looking down at my filthy clothes. I knew she was just being polite.

"No ma'am, but if you don't mind, I'll go out to the well and clean up just a little. Maybe I can get some of this dried material off my arms before Jan gets here."

"Well, I hope you and your family have a merry Christmas," she said.

Soon I was washing off with a bucket of cold water and scrubbing with a bar of Lava soap. I thought about how ridiculous the entire scenario was and how amusing regular people might find it. I laughed and shivered as I soaped and washed, then did it again, finally drying off with a large feed sack hanging nearby.

To escape the cold midnight wind gusting out of the northwest, I sat down on the ground near the southeast corner of the well house. With my arms crossed and held tightly to my chest, I felt relaxed and almost comfortable for the first time in several hours. I must have dozed off briefly because presently I heard a vehicle slowing down, then crunching on the gravel of the driveway just yards away. I knew from the sound it was Jan's station wagon. Never had I been so glad to see a warm car and friends.

"Oh, honey, I know you are freezing to death. I've got the heater all warm and everything. Are you OK?" It's nice to have a spouse who always responds positively to unpleasant situations.

The warm seats of the car felt so good and at that moment I thought I might even recover from the difficulties of the last several hours. When I looked around and saw the two little ones all bundled up and sleeping in the back, I knew things would be just fine.

Jan wanted to know all the details and as I related the events to her, I noticed she was covering her nose and mouth with the collar of her big coat.

"What's the matter?" I asked.

"John, you smell horrible! I think I'm going to be sick," she said slowly. "Reckon you could take those clothes off?" She has always had a weak stomach, even weaker than the coon hunters'. I realized she was only seconds away from suffering the same fate.

"Well, I guess so," I replied.

Quickly, I pulled the malodorous tee shirt over my head. Next came the khaki pants, shoes, and socks.

"Stop down here at Miss Ruby's store and I'll just put these clothes on the front porch, then pick them up tomorrow when I get my truck," I suggested.

Soon we were out on the main highway to Butler. I believe it was the first and only time I have ever ridden in a car attired only in pink jockey shorts. According to Jan, the bulk of the smell had disappeared with the outer garments. She was beginning to talk again, indicating that the nausea was easing off.

We were quietly discussing the day's events and tomorrow's chore of extracting the truck as we pulled into the Butler city limits. Even though the town was decked out in its Christmas finery, things were pretty dead, as usual.

When the traffic light turned red, Jan slowed down to stop.

"Run it, nobody's around," I declared.

"What if I get caught?"

"Run it! Walter's bound to be asleep!"

"OK, whatever you say." Then she eased on through, looking carefully both ways.

We had not gone a block when I saw bright lights coming up behind us and then the flashing red light began its eerie rotation.

"Oh no!" Jan exclaimed. "It's the law!" She pulled over and stopped by the drugstore.

"No, it's not, it's just Walter, the town policeman," I said, looking back and seeing the old white police car. Walter exited the car, adjusted his gunbelt, and put on his hat. Then he marched up and tapped on the car window, trying to look inside.

"Good evenin', ma'am. Could I see your driver's . . . uh, is that you, Miz Doc?"

"Yes sir, Mr. Walter, and I'm so sorry about running that light. It's sort of an emergency, you see. I had to get the kids out of bed to go pick up Dr. John, because his truck broke down up north of Lisman at Miss Ruby's, and . . ." She was on a roll and could have gone on and on, but then the flashlight beam was being trained on me. First my face, then the beam slowly traveled down my bare chest, then paused briefly at my shorts before going down to my legs to the floor.

"Doc John, why are you nearly nekkid? And what is that smell? Y'all ain't been over to them state-line beer joints have you?"

"Walter, just let us go on home and I'll come by City Hall tomorrow and explain it all to you. Then you'll understand. OK?"

"Uh, I guess that will be fine. But the mayor told me to stop anybody breakin' the law, didn't make no difference who it was!" he preached. The light was in my face now.

"Well, he didn't mean me. You know I'm out all hours of the night trying to heal the sick," I retorted. "I'll see you sometime tomorrow."

"Awright, Doc, I'll let you go this time. But while I've got you stopped, Doc, I've got this dog out at the house, and he's been coughin' real bad. Reckon it's worms? You remember I talked to you about him before, but he's got bad again."

"I'll see you tomorrow, Walter. I'm too dern tired to think." My eyes were closed, not so much from exhaustion as from the unrelenting flashlight beam.

"By the way, those sure are pretty shorts, Doc. Did you get 'em down at Bedsole's?"

"No, I got 'em at the J.C. Penney over at Meridian," Jan chimed. "They also have blue, red, yellow, and green, but as you can see, John likes pink. They're having a big sale on underwear all this week!"

"Let's *go!*" I bellowed. "This is *crazy!*"

It was only another half mile to the house, but it was a half mile of cheek-popping guffaws, loud enough to awaken the kids. Jan was having trouble driving, just thinking about the probable conversation at the City Hall the next morning.

"Guess who I stopped last night right here in town?" Walter would say.

"Who?" would ask Julia, the city clerk.

"Dr. John! Yeah, he was ridin' around after midnight with his good-lookin' wife, and she was all over the road and runnin' red lights. And get this! Doc was sittin' there buck nekkid, except for a pair of them little bitty pink tight shorts that don't hardly cover up nothin'!"

"You mean Dr. John the veterinary?"

"Yeah, the veterinarian! And you know what else? There was a bad odor in the car, too!"

"Uh oh! Bet they'd been drinkin' over at them state-line honky-tonks. They was all tanked up, I betcha. I didn't know Doc carried on like that, did y'all?"

Then everybody would shake their heads back and forth, even strangers who had come in to pay their utility bills.

By noon, talk would have reached Chappell's barbershop on the town square, and that was the Butler equivalent of the Associated Press. At Sunday preaching, a few of the holier-than-thou types would have their noses stuck straight up in the air when we met, attempting to punish me by not speaking.

That's all part of the excitement and challenge of living and working in a small town. I wasn't worried about the gossip as I showered and finally crawled into my bed that night. I was worried about how I was going to get my truck out of Miss Ruby's swampy pasture!

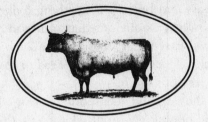

Chapter 16

I AWOKE WITH sunrise the next morning. My first thoughts were of my stuck truck and what I was going to do about it.

I was determined to try and extract the truck by myself. If I was unsuccessful, I'd have Jan take me back down to Jack Means's place and I'd borrow his tractor.

Soon Jan had Tom and Lisa up, dressed warmly, and fed, and we were retracing our steps of the night before. I was the driver this time and I obeyed each and every traffic signal and sign going through town.

"Why don't you just run that red light?" Jan urged, trying to stifle a giggle.

"I think not today. Walter might not be in a good mood this early in the morning. Besides, I'm not sure we need any more publicity after that deal last night," I replied.

A few minutes later we approached Miss Ruby's store and turned left onto the dirt road that led to her pasture. I could see my filthy clothes still there on the store's porch. I wondered what her morning customers would think, when they were greeted by such an unpleasant aroma.

"Do you want me to help, wait, or what?" Jan asked. "I could go ahead and take the kids to playschool."

"Yeah, why don't you do that. I'm sure I can get this thing out of there with a little digging. Take 'em on to school, then come back out here to be sure that I'm out and gone." With that I exited the car and went through the gap into the pasture.

It was only a two-minute walk down to where my truck sat, surrounded by tall grass and bushes. Everything looked so different in the light of day; now it was obvious that trying to drive in that area was a mistake. It was easy to see that it was a patch of low-lying area between two hillocks. The truck also appeared to have sunk deeper in the mud since the previous night.

I used my trusty shovel to dig out around the rear wheels and axle but the truck still would not budge. I figured, though, that if I could jump up and down on the rear bumper while the truck was in low gear, this up-and-down movement would extricate me from my muddy predicament.

I rigged up a remote-control device to the accelerator by using a horse twitch and some obstetrical wire. I jammed the twitch down on the accelerator and wedged it under the instrument panel so that the rear wheels would be in motion. Then I tied the wire around the middle of the twitch and ran it out through the open door. I reckoned that I could hold on to the wire and once the truck was moving forward, I would just jerk the twitch out from under the dash and the truck would stop, or at least slow down. If worse came to worst and it got to going too fast, I'd just leap through the open door. I congratulated myself on my dirt-road ingenuity.

After four or five strong jumps on the rear bumper, I was rewarded with success. The truck began to move. Suddenly, it lurched forward, throwing me off backward, and I lost my hold on the wire. Imagine my panic then, as my beloved truck started lumbering down the hill toward the biggest and deepest pond in all of Choctaw County while I frantically grabbed for the elusive wire. Never have I run so fast to catch up to a speeding and weaving object. Within seconds I was even with the rear wheels and gaining on the door, which had slammed shut.

Somehow, I managed to reach through the open window and grab the gear selector. Unfortunately, when I moved it upward it slipped into reverse, which quite effectively stopped the vehicle, but also bruised the transmission and damaged some of the motor supports. Miraculously, I found the truck could still run, and I was feeling right smug about my independence as I turned and drove along the edge of the pond.

But just as my newfound confidence was at its peak, I noticed the vehicle moving slower, and then failing to respond as I gave it more gas. It seemed to be sinking and there was nothing I could do except sit there and mash on the accelerator. I rocked back and forth a few times with no result. Then I discovered I couldn't open the cab door. I knew I was dealing with the grandma of all mired-up episodes.

"Now I'm worse off than last night!" I yelled. "Farther away from the gap, Jan gone, and I'm in mud so deep the door won't even open! Why didn't I take that fine job in Memphis?"

I was red-faced with anger at myself for my poor judgment. I should never have driven down that far in the pasture to start with. I should have gotten Jack Means's tractor the first thing that morning, and I shouldn't have let Jan leave until I was out in the road with my truck. I crawled out the window, fell in the thick, gumbolike mud, and tromped through the sage grass up the hill.

I was halfway to Miss Ruby's store when I heard a car roaring up the road. "Maybe it's somebody I know," I thought. "I sure hope so."

Sure enough, when the vehicle came around the curve, it was Jan's white Chevy station wagon. I have never been more pleased to see our own car!

"You're stuck again, aren't you?" she asked. "You got it out but then got into a deeper hole."

Jan has always had an eerie sense of clairvoyance. On several previous occasions she had sensed trouble when I was out making farm calls. Once I had walked into the house and she immediately asked about how bad I had been kicked. I had, in fact, been stomped rather severely by a high-spirited Tennessee walking horse.

"How did you know?" I asked, as I opened the passenger side door and flopped down.

"I don't know how, but I just felt something was wrong. I was just praying you weren't hurt. You aren't hurt, are you?"

"No, just mad at myself for getting into such a mess."

"Honey, you sometimes get so excited doing your duty, you go beyond what you ought to do. You really didn't need to drive your new truck way down in that pasture, did you? Couldn't you have stopped at the high ground near the gate?" she asked.

"But the cow was down there and I needed the light!" I replied. "Plus I'd have had to tote all my stuff down there."

"Maybe you should ask your clients to have their animals corralled or in the barn when you arrive. Wasn't that what that expert on veterinary practice management said in his lecture at the vet meeting this past summer?" she said.

"Aw, Jan, that guy is some smart Ph.D. professor from a veterinary school up North. He doesn't have any concept of the real world!" I bellowed.

"Well, I'll bet he's not stuck and all riled up to the point of a stroke," she said, sweetly.

"Jan, you don't understand! That guy doesn't understand! Nobody understands these farmers but me!"

"I understand you're fixing to blow a circuit if you don't calm down!" she replied, as we turned in at Jack Means's place.

Jack was a middle-aged farmer, originally from Cajun country down in Louisiana. He owned a herd of Santa Gertrudis and Brahman cows, a few horses, and a pen full of coonhounds. He also grew the usual assortment of farm crops. He was known as a good neighbor and always had a smile for everybody. He was in the backyard splitting wood when we drove up, and he stared hard at Jan's car, trying to figure out who it was.

"Mr. Means, I'm Dr. McCormack, the veterinarian. How are you today?"

Pleasantries were exchanged, the status of the cold weather discussed, and inquiries made about the family before the reason for my visit was made known. I then asked about the tractor.

"Sure, I'm not doin' anythin' important this mornin', so I'll go along and get you fixed up. As a matter of fact, I was gonna call you today. Got a sick cow down in the pasture," he said in his pleasant accent.

"It's sure nice of him to help, isn't it. Reckon what he'll charge you?" Jan declared, as we eased out the driveway.

"He won't charge anything. 'Course I'll doctor his cow for free. So I guess we'll call it even."

Jack's old putt-putt John Deere soon had the truck pulled out of trouble and back on the road, seemingly not much for the worse, except for a loose engine and a transmission that had a funny whine.

"I'll meet you at the barn, Jack, and we'll check that cow," I yelled as he came through the gap.

Ten minutes later Jack and I were carefully easing my muddy truck out into his pasture. I vowed to be very careful with it from then on.

No more mud hole challenges, no ripping through briars or small trees, and most important, no more fast driving.

"Doc, she's right over dere nex' to the bayou," Jack said in that south Louisiana accent. "Jus' drive down by dat live oak and you won't get mired up."

As we made our way down through the swampy pasture, I could see the old half-Brahman reclining, cow fashion, with her head crooked back on her side. When we passed under the oak tree she apparently heard us and her head shot straight up, like a periscope. I noticed right off that her head was quivering and shaking, and she looked as if she wanted to eat somebody, preferably an intruding veterinarian.

Then I noted the yellow color around her eyes and remembered the lecture on anaplasmosis I'd heard in veterinary school.

"By the time you are called, most cows will be exhibiting icterus," Professor Gibbons had said, "and they will be somewhat irritable. They will often be quite vicious and will charge and attack if provoked."

"Maybe you ought to ease over there and slip that rope over her head, since she knows you better than me," I suggested to Jack diplomatically.

He agreed, and slipped quietly out of the passenger side, eased over to her, and effortlessly dropped the lariat over her head. The cow kept shaking and staring right at me, only glanced once at her owner, and never offered to stand up.

The instant I detrucked and had both feet planted on the swampy pastureland, she immediately sprang to her feet and wildly bolted toward the figure now wearing *blue* coveralls and stethoscope. I jumped aside just in time to see her right horn and part of her head disappear into the lower portion of my door, accompanied by a tin-collapsing crash. My mouth was gaped open in shock and astonishment, and my eyes were riveted to the patient as she extracted her head from the truck door, staggered backward with eyes walled back in her head, and fell, graveyard dead amongst the mud and wet smutgrass.

"Doc, you killed my cow!" shouted an excited Jack, who was now jumping up and down on the poor beast's chest. He had probably read something about artificial respiration in a 4-H manual or the *Reader's Digest*.

After my fast-talking explanation of the pathogenesis of anaplasmosis, Jack appeared to accept that I was not the cause of her demise. As I recall, he told only about two hundred people about the event. He never mentioned anything about repairing my truck, though.

As I drove away from Jack's farm, I was shaken. Only hours before, I had driven a perfectly good truck, which someday would have been a collector's item for one of my grandchildren, into the McCord's Store area, only to damage the thing beyond the point of embarrassment. It was covered with mud, it whined and rattled, and now the driver's side door had a dent in it deep enough for a bird bath. As bad as I felt, there was one good thing. Thank goodness it was the truck and not the station wagon.

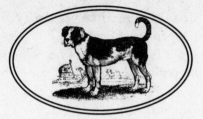

Chapter 17

ON CHRISTMAS EVE, we were frantically trying to get out of town to be with Jan's folks for Christmas. All the calls had been made, medications for ill ones dispensed, and our neighbors informed about our forty-eight-hour vacation. I was quickly loading the station wagon with essentials for the 150-mile trip, including the kids' Christmas presents.

As I secured the last of the toys onto the rooftop carrier, the sound of the telephone penetrated the semidarkness.

"Aw shoot!" I growled. "I was hoping we could get away before those after-six calls started."

Jan caught it on the third ring and shortly appeared at the back door.

"Telephone, honey!" she yelled. I could tell from the tone of her voice there was a problem. Frequently, I can get a pretty good indication of the caller's difficulty from the way she calls me to the phone.

She has a cow-in-labor tone of voice, a dog-hit-by-car tone, a possible-rabies-suspect tone, and still another distinct sound when there's someone on the line who wants to give us free cats or dogs.

"It's Mr. Hugh Jenkins," she said when I reached the door. "Why don't you see if it will wait until we get back."

I knew Mr. Jenkins, since I had recently gone by his house back in the hollow to vaccinate his pack of deer dogs against rabies. He was a brother of Carney Sam Jenkins, and the father of Joe Bob "Sinkin'" Jenkins, the famous fainter.

I was sure the present phone call related to a very serious animal health problem. Like most of his neighbors, Mr. Jenkins hated to spend money, so he delayed things like veterinary care and assistance until nature had been given every chance.

"Mr. Jenkins, what can I do for you?" I heard myself say.

"Zat chu, Doc?" he replied. I could hear the clicking of his store-bought teeth.

"Yessir, what's the matter?"

"Uh, it's Queenie, my main dog," he replied. It was obvious that he was uncomfortable talking over the neighborhood telephone. "She's been gone several days and just come up this evenin' with a bad hind leg. Looks like it's been hung up in a steel trap or somethin'."

"Is the leg cold?" I asked.

"Eh? How zat?"

"Cold! Is the leg cold?" I yelled.

I could hear mumbling and low talk on the other end. I reckoned that he was getting Joe Bob's thinking about the leg.

"Doc, Joe Bob says it was cold as a wedge when he checked it while ago," he answered.

"OK, I tell you what, Mr. Jenkins. We're on our way to Birmingham and we're coming that way. I'll be by there in about twenty minutes and take a look at her."

I'm sure that vet spouses sometimes get tired of "going by" to see patients when on their way out of town or coming home from church. However, it is often the most expedient thing to do, and sometimes it is the only thing that can be done short of canceling a long-awaited trip.

"Let's go! Let's go!" I repeated nervously as I herded Tom and Lisa toward the back door. Jan was plucking jackets, hats, and gloves off the coatrack with the speed and dexterity of a big-city magician. At the same time, I grabbed my emergency bags from the garage.

Minutes later we were buzzing out State Highway 10. Jan explained to the kids that Daddy needed to stop along the way for a sick dog and therefore the arrival time at Grandmother's house would be delayed.

Naturally, this news opened the floodgates to a barrage of questions. Even though they were both less than five years old, they were firing questions at me as if they were first-year vet students. They both wanted to assist with the examination and treatment, but I suggested that they would be of much greater benefit if they stayed in the car and listened to the radio.

Soon we were being jostled about as we slowly made our way up Mr. Jenkins's half-mile driveway. When I saw the dim light in a front window, I assumed that he had yet to show an interest in having the power company string a line up to his place. Therefore, a couple of kerosene lamps furnished the light that was needed for the household.

When we arrived in front of the old clapboard house, two figures tromped out onto the old rickety porch and eased down the concrete block steps. It was Mr. Jenkins and "Sinkin'" Joe Bob. One carried a lantern while the other was shining a flashlight up into the chinaberry trees, under the house, and right into our eyes. I figured it was Joe Bob playing with the light. That was the kind of thing he'd be doing, even though he was at least twenty years old.

"This way, Doc!" shouted Mr. Jenkins, just as I set foot on soil.

I followed the two men around the corner of the house where the cold northwest wind greeted my nostrils with the unmistakable scent of a well-populated nearby dog pen. The dogs exhibited their joy as we neared the pen by barking, whining, and leaping into the air. Some were jumping into the fence and biting at the gate hinges while others just stood, patiently wagging their tails and grinning. These grinners were actually pulling back their lips and showing their teeth in a joyful fashion.

"Queenie's over yonder under that lean-to," allowed Mr. Jenkins. "She's bad sick, Doc." I realized then that Joe Bob had yet to speak a single word. Instead he just kept on pointing the beam of the flashlight up into the trees, at stumps, and into my eyes.

Queenie was stretched out under the shelter on a pile of pine straw. When I spoke to her, she raised her head slightly, licked her lips, and cut her eyes upward until she was looking pitifully right at me. "Please help me!" her sad eyes seemed to be saying. From the looks of her frail and still body, she looked like she hadn't eaten or lapped water for at least a week.

Then I saw the leg. Her right hind limb, from just above the hock on down, was nothing more than a mass of gangrene. With such a terrible injury and in such a state of illness, I wondered why she was alive.

Unfortunately, the mutilated leg was a common type of injury seen frequently among deer dogs, coonhounds, foxhounds, and any other dog that ranged over long distances and jumped woven-wire or loose barbed-wire fences. The damage occurred when the dog attempted to jump the fence and one of the hind legs became entangled between the two top strands of wire. As the momentum of the dog carried it over the fence, the leg then became hopelessly entrapped in the twisted wire, leaving the poor beast hanging upside down. The animal might be there for an extended period until a Good Samaritan happened along or it someway managed to struggle free. In many cases, blood circulation to the lower leg was quickly interrupted, which resulted in a gangrenous and useless leg.

"Hold the light still, Joe Bob!" I fussed. "I'm trying to examine this leg!" But it only took a few seconds to palpate, squeeze, smell, and check for any signs of life in the affected foot.

"Can you help 'er, Doc?" Joe Bob finally asked as I slowly stood upright. I took a deep breath and commenced with the bad news.

"Well, we've only got two choices," I said. "Either we can put her to sleep or we can amputate that leg."

"You mean like take it off?" gasped Mr. Jenkins. I was glad that I couldn't see his face since it was no doubt bleached out and horror-stricken.

"But Doc, this is my best dog! She's a purebleed!"

The words had barely escaped his lips when I noticed that the flash-light beam was wobbling crazily; then I heard a soft, grunty groan from over to my left, followed quickly by a thunderous crash of some-thing heavy onto the doghouse over by the chinaberry tree.

"Joe Bob!" cried Mr. Jenkins. But there was no need to try to con-verse with Sinkin'. He was out, cold as kraut, lying belly down atop the doghouse roof.

"Here I am," I thought to myself, "out here on a cold Christmas Eve night trying to do the impossible. No light, a dog that's got to have a leg removed, burdened with a chronic collapser, spouse and children waiting on me out yonder in the car, and folks in the big city anxious about our whereabouts. In other words, a typical McCormack mess."

Mr. Jenkins was working on the immediate problem of getting Joe Bob to his feet and mobile. He rang his jaws two or three times, yelled his name, and fanned him with his hat. But alas, it was no use. Finally, in desperation, he filled a two-and-a-half-gallon zinc bucket of water from a full tub nearby and sloshed half of it directly into Joe Bob's face.

The deluge brought immediate results. Joe Bob came up sputtering and shaking his head as if he had ear mites. Almost as quickly as he had fainted, he was back on his feet, mumbling and blindly groping for his old flashlight.

"Wonder how come it is that he's all time doin' that?" Mr. Jenkins asked, gazing right at me.

"His stomach gene is weak, I guess," I replied. I wonder why he thought I'd know!

With Joe Bob resuscitated, we finally made a decision on Queenie. At the urging of Mr. Jenkins, I agreed to take off the leg. I would anesthetize her on the front porch and perform the surgery while standing on the ground.

While Mr. Jenkins brought our patient around to the surgical "suite," I ran to the car and informed Jan and the kids that I'd be at least another thirty minutes. Of course, they were ready to travel but they appeared to understand the problem. I retrieved my equipment from the back of the station wagon and quickly hoofed it back to the porch where Queenie had been placed.

While rummaging through the car I had found a light that could be attached to the user's cap. I had often used it when doing nighttime large animal work. I strapped it on to the front of my head, turned on the switch, and found that it worked nicely.

Presently Jan was at my side, arranging all my surgical equipment in convenient fashion while I went to work. After I gave the anesthetic, I shaved and cleaned up the surgical area, then washed my hands and gloved up.

Mr. Jenkins had seated himself in the porch swing just above us and to the right. During the surgery he nervously swung back and forth and amused himself by humming hymns and whispering prayers. Joe Bob had stumbled into the house and was resting on the daybed in the front room. I whispered a prayer asking that he stay there.

Everything went well and it wasn't long before I was putting in the skin sutures. Queenie looked as well as could be expected after her ordeal. After cleaning up and giving her antibiotics, we placed her on an old quilt and carefully carried her to the barn where we found an empty stall. We made a comfortable bed out of loose grass hay and then gently placed her down in the middle of it.

"She'll sleep for several hours," I told Mr. Jenkins, "but I think she'll be good and awake by morning." Then I explained how I wanted him to feed and water her the next day, plus how he should take care of the incision. I promised to come by and check on Queenie on our way home.

As we left the stall, he disappeared through the back door of the house while Jan and I cleaned up the instruments and put them back into the car.

"What do you think?" I asked Jan.

"Oh, she's a tough old dog," she replied. "I'm sure she'll do fine."

"I don't know, Jan. It was pretty crude, without proper sterilization, no intravenous fluids, no warm recovery area. I'm sure my vet school surgery professors would have had a runnin' fit if they knew I was using that front porch for a surgery table and a coon-hunting lamp strapped on to my head for a surgical light."

"Honey, you did the best you could with what you had to work with," she said. "You did a good job in a less than perfect situation."

By then, Mr. Jenkins had reappeared carrying a large box and a coin purse. It was one of those small leather purses that had two compartments and little metal latches at the top. He paid all his bills in cash, and tonight was no exception as he meticulously counted out the amount that I had requested into my hand. Then he handed me the mysterious box.

"Here's a little somethin' extry for y'all," he said sincerely. "Miz Doc, maybe you can fix the good doctor some of this for his breakfast. Thank both of y'all for what you did."

Inside the box was a country ham that he had cured himself. I had reservations about accepting such a nice gift when I knew he needed the money it would have brought in town, but it was obvious that he sincerely wanted to give us something more than my fee.

The trip back out the driveway didn't seem nearly as rough as it had an hour or so before. Jan and I were keyed up and feeling good about what we had accomplished, even though it was not something that would be earthshaking enough to even make the weekly Choctaw County paper. Still, it was almost guaranteed to be a big item at barbershops all over the area.

Being away from work for forty-eight hours at Christmastime isn't much of a vacation, but we crammed a lot of enjoyment with our family into that short period.

Christmas Day was spent with Jan's parents in Birmingham. Then right at nightfall we reloaded the station wagon and started the 120-mile drive to Tennessee for a short visit with my parents.

Some two to three hours later up the highway, we turned down the narrow driveway to the farm of my childhood. The lights of the station wagon pierced the darkness of the pasture adjacent to the gravel road and quickly encountered several cows standing beside the feed trough. Since their coats were black as coal, only their retinas reflected the light. The ghostly glowing eyes were the only visible evidence of cowhood on the hoof. All four occupants of the car stared in awe and amazement at the wonder of nature before us.

Soon we were being profusely but ungraciously greeted by Bingo, the old dog, whose warning barks quickly gave way to joyous jumping and nuzzling when his nose finally identified our scent as friend, not foe. Even though our trips home to the farm were months apart, old Bingo remembered us each time.

Seconds later, happy children were bursting through the back door into the arms of even happier grandparents, who were patiently looking from one child to the other as the miracle of the shining cow eyes was related simultaneously by the youngsters.

The familiar aroma of burning oak wood and my momma's kitchen was comforting and induced a state of contentment as we settled in. The roast beef on the stove, the four-layer cake covered with hand-grated coconut, made my mouth water, but nothing pleased my nose quite so much as her homemade rolls. None I have ever tasted since have matched hers for their yeastiness and country good flavor. Once as a teenager, I consumed eleven of those delicacies at one sitting, each having been daubed with a gob of real, hand-churned-by-the-fireplace butter.

Early the next morning I brought Mr. Jenkins's ham into the kitchen for my mother's inspection.

"Where did you get such a beautiful ham?" she exclaimed. "It looks like one of Frank's except not as big."

My uncle Frank was a master at salt-curing pork. He had a special box in the smokehouse in which he layered the fresh hams, shoulders, and side meat and then covered them in salt. Sometimes he added a little sugar for flavor and a little saltpeter to help maintain the nice pink color in the meat. The meat remained buried in the salt for varying amounts of time, depending on the cut of meat and its thickness. After several days of salt penetration, the juices oozed out of the meat as the curing process took place. The end result was preserved pork meat that needed no refrigeration, which after all was the reason for all the effort in the first place. The only problem with the meat is its high salt content, which is objectionable to some. Others like the briny taste. The salt content of the cured hams can be reduced by soaking them in clear water for a day or two before eating, but there was no time for that with Mr. Jenkins's donation.

Mother's big butcher knife sliced through the ham butt with ease. The quarter-inch slabs that flopped onto the cutting board were a beautiful pink color, encircled with a half-inch border of pure white lard. At the time, the word "lard" had not yet been exiled into the bad word category. That would come later, thanks to the all-knowing TV health reporter.

Later, as we breakfasted on fried ham, fresh eggs right from a hen-house nest, redeye gravy, grits, more butter, Momma's big cathead biscuits, and fresh raw milk from the Jersey out in the barn, I related the story of Jenkins's dog, being careful to leave out most of the goriness.

"You mean he actually paid you cash money to operate on the dog, plus gave you this ham?" exclaimed Dad, just before poking a double-bite-size chunk of ham into his mouth.

"Yes sir, that's right. But you need to understand that this was his main hunting dog," I replied.

He mumbled something about wasting time doctoring on dogs when there were cows and pigs out there dying. But he kept right on eating that fine ham. Dad never did have a lot to say, but that was all right. I knew that he and Mother were proud of what we were trying to do. To them, helping farmers and country folks was a calling of the highest order, and that is probably one reason I selected rural Alabama for a veterinary practice rather than Miami or Memphis.

It was all over too soon. Less than twenty-four hours later, we were repacked and buzzing southward.

We felt rejuvenated from the short contact with our loving and supportive families. They were excited about what we were doing and were always anxious to hear of our adventures, both good and bad, and how the practice was progressing. Even though we were full grown and parents ourselves, I knew they worried about us, so far away and in unknown territory. A couple of hundred miles seemed a lot farther back then than today, especially to my relatives, all of whom were living within a short distance of where they were born. I would find out when my own children were older that parents are always concerned about their offspring, regardless of their age, geographic location, or station in life.

We went by to see Queenie on the way back, and found that she was up and around on three legs, had eaten some table scraps and consumed a lot of water. I left more medicine for her and asked Mr. Jenkins to call if anything went wrong. When I went on about how much we all enjoyed the ham, he seemed mighty pleased.

Several weeks later, I saw him in town and he told me that Queenie was hunting at full speed and keeping up with the other dogs. Animals continually amaze me with their powers of convalescence.

I have thought about the Queenie episode and others like it many times over the years and I am not ashamed of the way I have handled them. Many times it is impossible to perform animal surgery in ideal conditions with all the proper instruments, drugs, and professional aftercare. More often than not, we are faced with challenges that include inclement weather, restraint problems, poor lighting, and fainting fellows like Joe Bob "Sinkin'" Jenkins. Even though no veterinarian prefers working under these conditions, overcoming these adversities and still getting the job done makes recovery back to production a satisfying event. You may even get a country ham!

Chapter 18

JANUARY 1964 STARTED off busy. Calving season was upon us, and the difficult-birth calls were increasing, along with the after-calving complications of vaginal tears, paralysis cases, and retained placentas.

Then there are the prolapses of certain portions of the reproductive tract. When veterinarians get together to tell war stories and tall tales, each one has at least one prolapse story to tell.

When an organ prolapses, it escapes from its normal position through a body opening and protrudes to the outside, highly visible for the rest of the herd or every nosy citizen of the county to see as they pass by. Body parts such as the vagina, cervix, and rectum can and frequently do prolapse, which creates an uncomfortable and dangerous situation for the animal, and a chore of moderate to severe difficulty for her doctor.

But the biggest prolapse of all occurs when the entire uterus of a cow, sometimes called the calf bed, decides to vacate its normal position. This is the mother of all prolapses. Even the greenest of cow observers knows at a glance that something is badly wrong when they see a washtub full of strange material hanging from the rear parts of a cow. Not only is the organ outside of the cow, it is also turned wrong side out.

"We won't never get that thing back in that cow," is the first thing a cattleman or cowboy will always say when observing a prolapsed uterus. That's why I was summoned on a January day.

I was fortunate to find the cow penned and waiting. That was unusual because the typical prolapse patient is still in the pasture getting the prolapsed organ dirtier and kicking at the long thing tickling her ankles. But it was covered with plenty of mud, straw, and other debris.

"I won't ever get that thing back in," I muttered when I first observed the huge swollen structure. After all, it was going to be necessary to stuff the whole mass back through an opening about one-tenth its size.

There is no way a person can be adequately instructed regarding uterine prolapse replacement. Although there are textbooks on the subject and helpful procedures such as spinal anesthesia and proper placement of the cow's hind legs, once the normal anatomical structures are understood the only way of learning how to accomplish the task is to just get down and do it.

The major problem, once an attempt is made at pushing and shoving the organ back inside the cow, is that the half ton of cow is better at pushing and shoving backward than a one-hundred- to two-hundred-pound human is at shoving and pushing forward. It becomes apparent very quickly that the cow doesn't want the offensive thing back inside her body. This is where spinal anesthesia may be helpful.

The key to success is perseverance, persistence, and pushing. Being ox-strong can be a decided plus, if that strength is used with caution and judgment. A sudden push could result in punching a large hole through the uterus, which does not improve the patient's chances for further offspring, and it tends to rile the farmer, who is usually sitting comfortably nearby.

I had two so-called assistants this day. One was a young lad of about fifteen. His main function seemed to be throwing up and going on about how gross the whole thing was. While he was evacuating his stomach over in the bushes, the elderly gentleman with him was trying to be helpful. Unfortunately, he was at least 103 years old, deaf, and with severely arthritic fingers. I knew he wouldn't be able to help much.

After washing and scrubbing the organ, the replacement effort began. While I shoved and massaged, I also constantly grunted, groaned, grimaced, and gasped for air. This action seems to help me make the gradual progress that is so encouraging.

Meanwhile, I heard the familiar questions from the onlookers.

"How's it comin', Doc. Havin' any luck?" I wondered why they always say that.

"It ain't goin' back in, is it, Doc?"

"You sho are gettin' nasty, Doc."

The proper response to the statements is a loud groan-grunt sound. Sort of a "Nawwyeahhhdonnomaybe" kind of vocalization.

"Can I do somethin' to he'p ye?" the nice old man asked.

"Naw sir, I think not," I mumbled, straining.

"How's that, sonny?" he yelled.

"NO!" I scream-grunted.

A few seconds later, I felt guilty about having hollered at the gentleman, so I decided to ask him to do something. Besides, I was having trouble.

"Get me a bar of soap!" I yelled.

"What ye want rope for?" he asked.

"*Soap! Soap!* A bar of *soap!*" I screamed. "So I can clean this thing up again and maybe I can get it to slip back in easier!" The kid was over by the gate, retching.

A few minutes later the gentleman returned from the back porch with a chunk of lye soap the size of a brickbat.

"You got any Ivory or Camay?" I asked.

"Do which?" he said, cupping both ears.

"Never mind! We'll make do with what we've got," I retorted, as I commenced a second scrub-down.

Lye soap is not the substance of choice for cleaning or lubricating a prolapsed uterus. Sometimes, though, you have to use whatever you have on hand.

Finally, after twenty minutes of straining, grimacing, and properly timed grunting, I could feel progress being made, even if it was only an inch at a time. I found that if I shoved a small portion of the organ back in around the edges just as the cow relaxed long enough to inhale a fresh breath of air, I could hold my position with both hands until she needed more air. Then I would repeat the process.

Just as total exhaustion seemed imminent, the uterus flopped back inside the cow and great sighs of relief were heard all around, even one from the bovine patient. There are few sights to a bovine gynecologist as sweet as the sight of the last twelve inches of a prolapsed uterus disappearing from view into the innards of an uncooperative patient.

But that's not the end of the job. The organ must then be straight-

ened out properly or it is apt to reprolapse. Imagine pulling your hand
out of a tight glove. As the fingers are withdrawn, the glove fingers are
also withdrawn, resulting in a totally inside-out glove. The hand portion of the glove can be replaced easily, but getting the fingers back in
proper position is more difficult. So it is with replacing a uterus. The
two horns must be manipulated into their normal anatomical position.

I was having difficulty getting the uterus to properly invert itself in
the present patient. The right horn was still balled up, and it was
almost out of reach. I could just touch it with my fingertips.

"Go get me a big bucket of water from the well, young man, and
hurry!" I declared. The kid didn't seem too bad off at the moment,
even though his face had taken on the coloration of pond water.

Minutes later, with bucket in hand and the boy watching, I attached
a large stomach tube to a pump, and then introduced the free end of
the tube deep into the cow's reproductive tract.

"Now pump!" I ordered.

"How?"

"Just take that handle, pull it up, then push it down. Reckon you
can do that?" I figured that it would be a challenge for him, but somehow he quickly got the hang of it.

As the water filled the uterus I felt it pop back into its proper position. I knew that after a couple of gallons had been pumped in, the
cow was going to do her best to send it back out.

"OK, that's good. Now move back because she's gonna send it back
out as soon as I move my arm."

Sure enough, the instant I extracted my arm, she strained, gushing
a stream of reddish-colored water some six to eight feet backward,
drenching the young man's white tennis shoes.

"Oh, gross!" he cried, while trying to escape the sudden torrent.
"My shoes are ruint!"

"Naw, they'll be OK. Just wade through the branch on the way
home and that'll take care of the red color and the smell too," I
declared, trying not to laugh. Anybody who would wear white shoes
to such an event needed to have them soiled.

After the cow had evacuated all the water, I dropped some antibiotic boluses into the uterus and put a couple of sutures across her rear
parts, just in case the idea of a repeat performance crossed her mind.

The old man had said little until I started my washup. But then he began to ask the usual questions about the aftercare of the cow and her future as a breeder and whether or not he should keep her.

"I'd keep her up close for a few days so you can pay close attention to her just in case she might reprolapse. If she's a good cow I'd suggest keeping her, because a prolapse of the uterus won't often happen again the following year," I yelled.

Soon he was pulling the greenbacks from his double-pocketed coin purse and placing them carefully in my open palm, one by one. I wondered if he would have enough to pay my fee and still have a little left over. I knew it was hard for an old person on a fixed pension to come up with money for unexpected expenses, such as an animal emergency, and I felt a little guilty having to ask him for money. But I was trying to run a business, and I had expenses too, plus a family at home who needed financial support.

"What do ye do for a livin'?" he asked as I stowed my gear in the truck. I was taken aback by the question.

"Why, I doctor on animals, both large and small," I answered.

"Naw, I mean what is yo' regular day job?"

"Doctoring animals is what I do for a living full-time. I don't have another job."

"So you are a full-time vetran."

"Yes sir, that's right. A full-time veterinarian," I repeated.

"Well, I shoulda knowed that by the way you charged," he replied, looking down into his flattened purse.

I looked in the rearview mirror as I drove away, and saw the cow picking up bits of straw and hay off the barn lot ground. Her tail was raised and I noticed her looking back at her rear end, obviously wondering what had just happened there.

Then I noticed the old gentleman standing by the fence. He too was staring, but first at the cow, then down at his coin purse, probably wondering what had just happened *there*.

On my way home from the exhausting prolapse replacement ordeal I decided to stop for a haircut and some conversation at Chappell's barbershop.

Chappell's barbershop was a three-chair establishment some twelve feet wide and nearly thirty feet long. The barber chairs were equally spaced along the left side and a long bench lodged itself against the right wall. On both sides were long mirrors which served as an entertainment feature. It always gave me an eerie feeling to stare into one of the mirrors, seeing my image being reproduced over and over again, smaller and smaller, fading into infinity. Any head movement would result in an identical response by the endless queue of curly-headed clones waiting for their appointment under the barber's scissors.

On my previous trips to the barbershop, I had found it was a great place to catch up on all the local, regional, national, and international news and events. If you sat there long enough you would see nearly everybody, because they would either pass by on the big road and wave or they'd come in for news or a haircut. You could also hear the latest sports predictions, learn about the potential severity of the upcoming winter, and find that among the barbers and those waiting to be clipped there were several individuals who were self-appointed authorities on one or more subjects.

One subject discussed frequently in the shop was Alabama football. Not the status of the sport in the state, but rather the football fortunes of the University of Alabama. The state's other class 1-A team, Auburn—my alma mater—was discussed minimally, because it was located way across the state and it wasn't winning as many games as Alabama.

Like the vast majority of Alabamians, I too enjoyed college football, but I was amused at the perceptions some of the barbershop sitters held. Some were card-carrying alumni of the university, a few had children attending there, while others were what I called "sidewalk" alumni. They mostly pulled for the team that was winning the most games any given year. Many of these sidewalk alumni had never been any closer to the campus than viewing a picture of the stadium in the weekly newspaper.

"Doc, did you go to college?" a sitter had asked the last time I was in the hair chair.

"Got my degree at Auburn," I proudly stated.

"Well, y'all have a pretty good team," he replied. "Got a fairly good coach and the stadium's real nice." This was a typical condescending remark uttered by a typical sidewalk Alabama alumnus. He really thought he was being complimentary.

"Oh yeah, we've got a fine library, a top-notch veterinary college, and there's all sorts of egghead, Ph.D. professors wandering around the campus trying to remember where they parked their bicycles."

"But how many games will they win this fall? Reckon they can give Alabama a game?" was the obvious response to my asinine reply.

"I hope they can, but the main thing is academic achievement, isn't it?" I knew I was making dangerous statements, suggesting that athletic entertainment was a secondary endeavor.

The sitter stared at me as if he couldn't fathom the strange ideas that he had just heard. What was wrong with this vet? Did he just get kicked in the head by a mad mule or something?

But today, I was hoping that the "sidewalkers" would be at the drugstore or feed store, harassing the customers there. Perhaps I would only have the world experts to deal with.

"Looka yonder who's coming through the door, Chappell. It's supervet hisself!" cried Myatt, cutting hair in the middle chair. Because Chappell was hard of hearing, he was in charge of the third chair, which was closer to the radio. The first chair was unattended except for Friday and Saturday, when a part-time preacher was called in to help out.

Myatt always referred to me as "supervet" whereas Carney Sam Jenkins was just called "vet." I appreciated being elevated to a higher standard than the local unlicensed competition.

"What you been up to this morning, Doc?" questioned Chappell.

"Aw, he's been out runnin' over dogs and sowin' hog cholera virus," instantly replied Myatt, never looking up from the head of hair he was demolishing.

The three bench-sitters sniggered and snorted their approval.

"Actually I just put in a prolapsed uterus over at Pushmataha," I declared.

"You put sugar on it?" asked one of the sitters, putting aside the antique and dog-eared *Sports Illustrated* magazine he was reading. No doubt he was trying to find a picture of the Alabama football stadium.

"Sugar?" Myatt replied.

"Yeah, sugar."

"For what?" Chappell asked.

"Well, Carney Sam does it. I saw him do it with my own eyes," said the sitter. "He took a five-pound sack of Domino's sugar, poured it over that calf bed, then rubbed it in. It went back in too, slick as a whistle."

"Naw! What does puttin' sugar on it do, Doc?" someone asked.

"Makes it sweet. And it's got to be Domino's, 'cause no other brand works!" I replied, straight-faced as an undertaker.

This brought forth several hoots, and a loud snort from Myatt. Chappell's shaving victim tried to laugh from his prone position, but with a straight razor poised at his throat by a jumpy barber he dared not move anything north of his Adam's apple. I could see his paunchy belly jumping up and down as he tried his best to stifle his mirth.

"What actually happens," I went on, "is the sugar draws fluid out of the edematous organ through osmosis, and that reduces its size, which makes it go back in the cow easier, don't you see."

The crowd was now silent, as if trying to assimilate the information they had just received. Finally, the customer in Myatt's chair spoke.

"Oz *what*?"

"Osmosis. Remember in high school chemistry when you learned that fluid will cross a membrane from a lesser concentration to a greater concentration? That's the principle involved."

I should have known the word "chemistry" would put the quietus on the conversation. Sometimes just hearing the words "chemistry," "physics," or "zoology" gives science haters the heebie-jeebies.

"It's been a long time since I fooled with chemistry," yelled Chappell. "I don't remember that much . . ."

"Aw, Chappell, chemistry hadn't even been invented yet when you were in school," Myatt declared in his best insulting tone. He winked and shook his head at his audience. Chappell finished shaving his patient, oblivious to Myatt's discourtesy and the guffawing of the crowd.

"Next!" cried Chappell.

"Go ahead, Doc, we ain't in no hurry," said one of the sitters. "I know you got things to do, dogs to operate on and all . . ."

I eased into the chair. Chappell popped the big hair-catching towel, then tightly pinned it around my neck.

"When he said operating on dogs it reminded me of something, Doc," he said. "The other day, Mr. Jimmy Throckmorton was sittin' right here in this chair and we was talking about you. He said after watchin' you operate on his prize dog, he thought you was the best surgeon in this county, by far."

"Really! He said that?"

"Yeah. And you know Dr. Perry, that surgeon we got over yonder over at the hospital, don't you?"

"Uh huh, we've heard he's real good."

"Well, Dr. Perry was sittin' right over yonder on that bench, reading the paper and smokin' that Chesterfield cigarette. When Mr. Jimmy made that statement about you, I thought Dr. Perry was gonna bite that cigarette in two! His face turned red as a rooster's comb."

"What did Dr. Perry say?"

"He didn't say a word, just buried his head in the newspaper and puffed harder on that cigarette."

"Mr. Jimmy ought not of said that. You know he exaggerates everything."

"Yeah, but he thinks a lot of you. He said if he ever got sick, he'd just as soon have you as anybody. And as hard as it is to get a doctor around here, it might even come to that."

"I hope not. Mules and cows don't complain at all when you doctor on 'em. They just kick, butt, or bite. But people carry on too much about a little pain," I declared.

In spite of all the useless chatter, know-it-all characters, and hypnotizing mirrors, the barbershop still remains one of my favorite loafing sites. The country barbershop is the equivalent of a thirty-seven-item insult bar. The barber keeps your hair from getting too long, and the bench-sitters keep your head from getting too big.

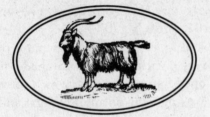

Chapter 19

WHEN I ARRIVED home from the barbershop, there was an ugly car parked out front. It was a dark gray four-door Dodge sedan, devoid of chrome, whitewall tires, radio, or any other niceties.

As I looked over the dull auto, I spied the U.S. Government license tag, which caused me immediate consternation. Like most good citizens, I become slack-jawed and stammer-lipped when faced with a visit, letter, or phone call from an unknown official of the government.

But when I parked and walked by the car, the stern lettering on the driver's side front door gave me immediate relief. In bold letters it read, "United States Department of Agriculture, Animal Research Service, Animal Disease Eradication Division." Underneath the big letters were a series of smaller letters, possibly the initials of a lesser division of government, the meaning of which was unknown to all but an occasional informed taxpayer or retired government worker.

To Choctaw Countians, the sighting of such an automobile would carry no specific significance, other than the fact that it was being driven by just another "govmunt leech" who filled his days by riding all around the countryside, wasting gas, wearing out tire rubber, and attempting to appear official.

"John, this is Dr. Stewart from the USDA in Montgomery. He has come to help get us started on the brucellosis testing in the county," Jan declared.

"Yes, we met at the cattlemen's meeting back in November," I allowed, shaking his hand.

"Good to see you again, Dr. John. We in Montgomery are so glad you are here in this county. We didn't know how we were going to get all the cows tested over here."

Dr. Stewart looked more like a retired senator than a government veterinarian. He wore a dark gray suit, starched white shirt, quiet tie, and black wing-tipped Sunday slippers, which carried the shine of an office worker. He was chewing on an unlit cigar and toyed with an Al Capone hat as he talked.

"First, I want to fix you up with some supplies," he stated, lifting a large cardboard box onto the coffee table. "Here are ear tags of all kinds that you'll need, blood tubes, needles, tagging pliers, and all the proper forms." He quickly flipped through a twelve-inch stack of papers.

"Here's the ADE 1-23 form, the ADE 3-59F, 33-01, ADE 1-27, and all your vouchers to fill out after you complete the blood-testing at each farm." Then he reached deeper into the box and retrieved another stack. "These are your quarantine notices, test charts, and finally, a copy of the Uniform Methods and Rules for the program."

"You mean I've got to fill out all those forms?" I whined.

"That's correct. But of course you won't have to fill out the quarantine notice, appraisal form, eradication plan, the ADE 1-27, or the ADE 1-23 unless you have positive reactors on any given farm, don't you see," he exclaimed. "Of course you know it will be necessary to red-ear-tag the reactors and "B" brand them on the jaw. Then just be sure your paperwork gets to Montgomery in ten days to two weeks."

"What have I gotten into?" I thought to myself. "The only thing I hate more than filling out government paperwork is having to eat cooked oatmeal!"

"Don't worry, honey, I've got it all written down. Dr. Stewart told me exactly which forms to fill out and when. Also, he showed me how to fill out the vouchers to get paid!"

Good old Jan! She not only was highly organized and efficient, but she could read my mind like a book.

"Second, I want to go over how you should approach these farmers to get them to agree to pen their cows up and allow you to test them," Dr. Stewart declared.

"Yes sir, I'd like some pointers," I confessed.

"What area of the county do you want to start in?"

"I haven't thought about an area. I figured I'd start with some of the cattle owners that I have met and worked for, because they are aware of the testing program," I replied. "Plus they want to get on with it and get their testing done this winter while it is easier to get their cows corralled."

"I'm afraid that's not how it's done. The government prefers that you divide the county up into various sections, then concentrate on those sections one at a time, going down the road in an orderly fashion."

That would be more difficult, as it required a lot more cold-calling on people who weren't aware of the program. Besides, I didn't want to be orderly about it!

"It seems to me that if I test the cows at the farms that I already know, those farmers will spread the word to the other owners in the area," I argued.

"I'm sorry, John. The official policy is as I have stated. Now which area of the county do you want to concentrate on first?" He unrolled a county map onto the coffee table and began scanning various roads, which were dotted with little black boxes, which I assumed represented houses.

"Why don't we divide the county into four quadrants. You have Highway Seventeen from north to south splitting the county in half, then Highway Ten from east to west," Stewart said.

"OK, let's do this section first," I declared, pointing to the southeast quadrant. "And let's start right here on Red Springs Road." I knew there weren't a lot of cattle down that road, but nearly every family owned a few. Perhaps the word would spread quickly since there were so many of the small farms to visit.

"Well, if you have a few minutes, let's run down there now and I'll make some appointments for you. That way you can see the proper way to initiate contact."

I wasn't sure that Dr. Stewart knew how to talk with the natives down Red Springs Road. These were very private people, who eked a living off the land by cutting timber, raising a few cows and pigs, and growing most of their own food. They were very close to their neighbors, yet they were resentful of strangers and outsiders. This was not the big cow country of Montgomery or Selma, and I believed Dr. Stewart would be met with stiff resistance if he used Washington bureaucrat talk instead of south Alabama logic.

These thoughts weighed on my mind as we motored the few miles southward in the discomfort of the government-issue sedan. Dr. Stewart was a careful, ultraconservative, and highly irritating driver. He kept tightly gripping and regripping the steering wheel and constantly shifting his hind end, apparently seeking the comfort channel worn in between the springs and padding of the seat by miles of driving. His head was constantly moving in all directions, peering into the rearview mirror, carefully reading roadway signs, and obeying each one to the letter.

But the most annoying feature of his driving was his erratic use of the accelerator. There was no continuity to our forward progress because of his constant jackrabbiting forward for several seconds, then falling back to turtle speed.

Then there was the cigar problem. He fired the thing up as we left the house, but after a few puffs, in between his advisory comments, it went out, and he spent the rest of the trip trying to strike matches and relight the offensive stogie.

By the time we turned off Highway 17, I was agitated, scared, and almost nauseous from tobacco fumes and abnormal auto motion. I was relieved when he stared at the first driveway and slowed to turtle speed.

"There's a few cows over there," he exclaimed. "Let's go see if we can get 'em lined up."

The residence was an old trailer house half hidden back in a grove of pine trees. At the sound of tires on gravel, two cur dogs came scrambling out from under the trailer, loudly announcing the arrival of the intruders. When they arrived carside, it became immediately apparent that they were in a vile mood. Even uneducated curs dislike ugly government cars.

"Not very friendly, are they?" Dr. Stewart said.

"No sir, I don't believe they've ever seen anybody from as far off as Montgomery before," I stated, trying to keep a straight face.

As I smiled at my elementary humor, the dogs vigorously attacked the slow-rolling wheels, snapping and biting at the tires as if they were some sort of whirling enemy invader. At least something was getting my mind off the disturbing antics of the driver.

We pulled up behind an old Chevy pickup that was decorated with a Confederate flag in the rear window and a bumper sticker that proclaimed, "This truck insured by Smith and Wesson." There were a couple of wrecked cars up on concrete blocks out near the privy, and junk of all description was scattered among the weeds and rusty barbed wire of the pasture fence line. A quick glance at the front of the trailer revealed a large overalled man standing just inside the open doorway. He was not smiling, and I sensed that his mood matched that of his dogs.

"*Shep! FIDO!*" he bellowed. Instantly, blessed quiet descended upon the scene. Even the echoes from the tall pines seemed to abruptly cease, obviously fearful of the big Bubba in the doorway.

"Uh, Dr. Stewart, I'm not sure this is such a good idea," I stammered. "Reckon we ought to go on to the next place?" I did not have a good feeling about this first stop.

"Nonsense! Those dogs won't bite. See, they're back under the mobile home." I noticed he said "mobile home." I made a mental note to practice saying that instead of "trailer house."

"Dr. Stewart, I'm not concerned about the dogs. It's that big-bellied guy standing yonder in the door," I said quietly.

"John, that guy puts his britches on just like the rest of us. Don't let anybody intimidate you, because you are now a representative of the U.S. Government!"

"Yeah, that's what worries me," I mumbled to myself.

Just seconds later, we were standing on a rickety stack of concrete blocks that served as makeshift steps to the trailer door. I was a couple of steps behind Dr. Stewart since he was going to do all the talking, which was fine with me.

"How're you today, neighbor?" exclaimed Dr. Stewart, without removing the Al Capone hat from his head. "I'm Dr. Stewart from Montgomery."

"Oh no, don't call him neighbor!" I silently screamed to myself. "And show some respect by taking off that hat. And why did you have to tell him you were from Montgomery?"

Most rural folks I know hate to be called "neighbor" by someone who is *not* their neighbor. They instantly know the guy is getting ready to cheat them out of something. My father never liked to be called "neighbor," especially by someone wearing an Al Capone hat.

"I'm awright," replied the resident, never uncrossing his arms from their perch atop his plenteous paunch. I knew right off from the way his mouth turned down at the corners and his bottom jaw jutted out that he was going to offer stiff resistance to anything we might say from then on.

"Pretty day for January, isn't it?"

"I've seen better."

"What I'm here for, neighbor, is to offer you an opportunity to have your cows tested for brucellosis, a highly contagious disease of the bovine species. We can do this absolutely free, at no cost to you whatsoever. All you have to do is get 'em up in your barn over there," Dr. Stewart stated.

"What's in it fer me?" the guy said, still moving no part of his anatomy except his lips. His eyes didn't even blink. "They ain't nothing wrong with my cows."

"Well, you don't know that. It'll take a blood sample from them to find that out. Actually, we're requiring all cows in the county to be tested."

I remember wishing he hadn't said that. Now things were really going to get crossways.

"On whose authority?" the man asked.

"On the authority of the U.S. Government!" replied Dr. Stewart forcefully.

"You work for the govmunt?"

"I sure do."

Only then did the cow owner make a move. He unfolded his arms and with his right hand slowly reached behind the door and produced a double-barreled shotgun, which he pointed toward the ceiling.

"Then git y'all's se'f off'n my property!" he said firmly, but in the same tone of voice.

For a man some forty years my senior, Dr. Stewart sure could move fast! He half fell down the blocks, pushing me aside as he broke for the car.

"Good day sir, we won't be troubling you any more today," he said, now taking long plow mule–following strides. I was about halfway to the car when the man yelled.

"Hey, Red! Come back here a minute." I've been called "Red" all my days, especially by those who can't remember my name.

"Yes sir," I answered, stopping dead still.

"Don't I know you from somewhere?" he asked, still holding the shotgun but now pointing it to the ground.

"I'm Dr. McCormack, the veterinarian up at Butler," I replied, hoping my face wasn't too ashen and my voice wasn't shaking.

"That's right! I knowed I knowed ye!" he exclaimed, pointing a finger in my direction. "Stay right there for a minute."

Dr. Stewart was sitting in his car, lighting a new cigar. If his nerves were bothering him, he didn't show it.

"What do you think of this?"

I turned to see a beautiful puppy in the arms of the man. His coat was shiny and healthy, and his tail was wagging with great intensity.

"What a fine dog, so healthy-looking and obviously smart," I said, stroking the soft fur with a nervous hand.

"Yeah, belongs to my daughter. You gave him a blood transfusion right after you moved to Butler last November. You saved his life, Doc!"

"I'll declare! It's Peanut!" I rubbed the puppy's head and made all the routine mouth, eye, and skin checks for signs of good health. "Yes sir, I do remember that evening. You're Mr. Moseley, aren't you?"

"That's right. You sure got a good memory. By the way, Doc, we'll test them cows whenever you want to. And if you want me to, I'll see everbody on this road and get them lined up the same day. But looka heah, you better send that man with the suit and tie on back to Montgomery. Tell 'im we ain't foolin' with nobody from the govmunt."

At the end of the driveway, Dr. Stewart turned back toward town.

"Don't you want to visit some more farms?" I asked.

"Uh no, I really need to get on back to Montgomery before dark. I have some matters there that need my attention."

"OK. I think I can handle it now."

"John, what did you and that crazy fellow back there talk about?"

"Oh, I just bragged on his dog real big," I said. "I think it's real important to say nice things about a farm family's dog in this county, especially if you want to test their cows. He said I could test his cows anytime, and he'd be my lineup man down this road."

"Well, I'll declare, John. You did good! Did he say anything about me?"

I just said, "I don't think he cared for your hat much."

Dr. Stewart didn't crack a smile, but he did mash on the accelerator with increased intensity and chewed harder on his smelly cigar. We made the trip back into town in half the time.

"I reckon I'll just go back home and leave this area to you. Looks like you've made a good start at it. Just remember, do it in an orderly fashion."

"Plus don't wear a suit and tie," I thought. "And never, never admit you are associated with the govmunt!"

Dr. Stewart was actually a big help to me in carrying out my cow-testing work in Choctaw County. He visited with us regularly, brought supplies, and offered advice. But he never did offer to visit any more farms for the purpose of lining up work for me.

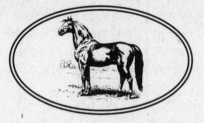

Chapter 20

PERHAPS THE MOST interesting thing about a general veterinary practice in a small town is its diversity. In a day's time a veterinarian might be called to perform a bovine obstetrical operation, diagnose the cause of lameness in a horse, repair a fractured femur in a dog, or treat diabetes in a cat. A county commissioner might call about a rabies problem in an outlying community, or a high school student could come by, seeking information and advice on her big science project.

In the first months of my new practice, I was surprised at the number of people who called asking for help with "exotic" animals. I would have preferred that one of my colleagues handle the health problems of fish, pet birds, gerbils, and raccoons, but since there were no colleagues in the area, I felt obliged to do my best to deliver the requested service.

However, there was another problem, and that was a matter of personal competency. Nearly all my professional training had been with farm animals and regular house and yard pets. In veterinary school there had been a few lectures and labs on the exotics, but at that time, veterinary knowledge of the wildlife species and unusual companion animals was lacking. There was little known about chemical restraint and drug dosages or how to physically handle them without endangering the lives of both patient and doctor.

I had seen a few monkeys as patients and I did not find them at all engaging, nor did they respond well to my treatments. It always took half a football team to restrain and examine a sick one and the other half had to hold legs and divert snapping teeth when the inevitable needle made contact with touchy monkey skin. Each time I participated in a monkey scrimmage, I prayed the next one to take sick in my territory would mercifully find some other animal-doctor victim somewhere who was more in tune with primate medicine and psychology. Finally, during my first months in Butler, I answered my last monkey call.

"Oh, please hep' me, Doctuh," the trembling voice pleaded over the phone. "It's my pet monkey."

"What's wrong, ma'am?"

"Oh, he's hung up high in a big live oak tree out front here and he can't get down. Oh, I'm so worried." I could hear sniffing, and the sounds of tear-mopping tissues being extracted from the box.

"Well, I suspect he'll climb on down when he gets hungry, don't you reckon?" I knew what was coming next, and I was killing time, trying to figure out ways to avoid climbing that tree.

I'll just admit it outright. I'm deathly afraid of high places. Lots of people have fear of heights, but I think mine is much greater than most.

If one of my best dairyman clients told me that a sick cow was perched atop of his eighty-foot-tall silo and that I was going to have to treat her there, I'd just have to turn in my calf jack and resign. He'd have to find someone else to climb up there. But the sniffing and Kleenex jerking was escalating into full-blown boo-hooing, obviously perfected over a lifetime of practice.

"I'm just an old shut-in lady, sick, nearly blind, and I don't have a dollar to my name. The only thing I have in this world is Monkey. Oh, what will I do?" I was sure her end of the phone line was dangerously soaked by then because of her overactive tear glands.

Naturally, being a Southern gentleman, I was unable to say no to a lady's entreaty. It didn't occur to me at that time, but since then I've often wondered why she didn't call the county agent, the volunteer fire department, or a professional coon hunter. Why the vet?

When I arrived at the address the lady had given, I found her out in front of her mobile home, wringing her hands and pointing animatedly up into the bowels of what surely was the largest live oak tree in the entire state of Alabama. If she could see a monkey in amongst all that foliage, she surely wasn't half blind. Then I noticed all the jewelry. Rings adorned every finger, bracelets and watches were rattling around on her wrists, and there must have been several pounds of gold and beads encircling her neck.

I've often wondered why it is that clients calling for urgent veterinary assistance are sometimes rather loose with the facts. So when a farmer calls and swears he has twenty cows dead and dying, I'm a little skeptical. And when pet owners who claim to be poverty-stricken and unable to pay a vet bill are decorated in expensive jewelry, I wonder if they have any concern at all for other people.

I climbed the tree, like an idiot, accompanied by a burlap sack. My plan was to get the monkey into the sack some way, tie it up with the twine I had in my back pocket, and make the lady happy. Looking back, I have no idea why I thought I'd ever be able to trap a monkey in a sack. At that moment I would rather have been trapped in the midst of a group of loose-boweled Brahman cows grazing lush clover in April.

I'd get up to him, only to see him bare his teeth and jump higher, just out of my reach. This went on for about twenty minutes. Finally I had gotten up into slender branches that could barely support my weight.

"Ma'am, I'm afraid that I'm not going to be able to catch him," I called down.

"Oh, no," she sobbed, "he'll die out here all alone. I love him so much, can't you just go out on that limb a little more? I just know you're going to get him this time." Why do women use this type of phrase on men so much?

I sighed and wished for those loose-boweled Brahmans as I inched forward another three feet. The monkey grinned like a dog with lockjaw, jumped higher, then made a few apelike grimaces.

At that point, I made the mistake of looking down. I was so high up in the tree the lady appeared to be a little dwarf about two inches high. No paratrooper in the army's history had ever been as frozen at the jump door as I was to that live oak limb at that instant. I cleared my throat, then spoke in as calm a voice as I could manage.

"Ma'am, I'm afraid to move. I've got myself way out here on this limb and I can't get back. You'll have to call the fire department in town and see if they can get me down," I said.

"Oh, oh, but what about Monkey?" she exclaimed. "He'll die!"

I won't repeat what I said at that point. It was neither nice nor professional, nor was it the kind of thing you should say to elderly ladies or clients. However, I do believe that there are times when the Master readily forgives us. I hope this was one of those times.

The poor lady clutched her hands to her gaping mouth, then turned and flew into the mobile home. Shortly, I heard her conversing loudly with a fire department member, and giving every detail about how many bodies were hung up in the tree. She also made it very clear that the "hung-up" human had not helped with her problem in the least, and poor Monkey was still up there, just minutes from certain extinction.

In about four hours, or maybe it was four minutes, I could make out the distant sounds of a whole covey of sirens. It wasn't long before I could see the rescue squad, the fire truck, a police car, and a deputy sheriff, all speedily bearing down on the scene at the big tree. All of the rescuers were grinning like possums as they detrucked and pointed fingers at the guy in the gigantic oak. I could hear them cackling like a flock of white leghorns, all of whom had just laid double-yolkers.

"Izzat you up 'ere, Doc?" one grinning paramedic-type uttered in between guffaws.

"Which one's the monkey?" another one cracked. Immediately, all hands roared as if they had been goosed in the ribs.

I slowly and carefully looked upward to the heavens for some blessed relief, only to see the stupid monkey baring his teeth and nonchalantly scratching his belly.

As I stared at the prissy primate, the limb to which I was glued seemed to suddenly drop, like a broken elevator. It was only the natural swaying of the branch in the breeze, but it made me catch my breath quickly and hold on even tighter. The laughing continued.

At that moment, I was too scared to be embarrassed. However, when I finally climbed down that fire truck ladder and set foot on firm soil, my feeling of relief was matched only by my humiliation. What could I do but thank all the volunteer firemen, get in my pickup, and let it whisk me away. I could feel my face burning and I knew that before nightfall, every Tom, Dick, and Bubba in the Southeast would know of the monkey episode.

Sure enough, the next morning I found a box on the front steps of my house. Inside were six packs of peanuts and a note:

For your monkey. You can have some too while
you are resting in the tree.
THE MONKEY PHANTOM

From that day on, I have avoided monkeys. When one comes in the front door for treatment, I hit the back door running, screaming, "It's an emergency! Bloated cow!" Whether that lady's monkey ever came down out of the tree is unknown to me. I confess I haven't spent a great deal of time worrying about it.

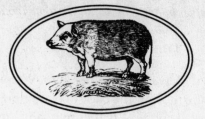

Chapter 21

A FEW DAYS after the monkey fiasco, I received a call presenting me with an opportunity for some skunk surgery. I instantly felt blessed, because dealing with anything besides a monkey was a step in the right direction. I even possessed a little medical and surgical experience regarding skunks.

"Is this Mr. McCormack, the venereal?" the female caller inquired.

"Yes ma'am, this is the veterinarian," I replied, trying to pronounce the *V* word very precisely, in hopes that she would remember it the next time. But I knew it was unlikely that she would get the message. I was indeed fortunate that she called at all.

"Well, Dr. Carney Sam Jenkins said I ought to call you about these baby skunks we found." Now Carney's a doctor and I'm a venereal!

"Skunks?" I replied. "Dr. Jenkins?"

"Uh huh, skunks. Dr. Jenkins said he was just so busy he couldn't help me with 'em and maybe you could. But he said you could use his shop for the operation."

"I see." That lying Carney! He knew even less about exotic animals than I did! He obviously didn't want to deal with the present situation so he was simply passing the buck, or in this case, the skunk, by claiming he was too busy.

"How much do you charge to fix a skunk?" she then asked.

"I don't believe that I've ever neutered a skunk," I replied. "Nor am I sure that I want to get into that."

"No, I mean fixing a little 'un so he won't smell bad. You know, doin' away with them stink glands."

"Oh, you mean a descenting operation," I answered. "We get twenty-five dollars for that."

"That is for the whole litter, isn't it?"

"No ma'am. That is per skunk," I replied boldly. "Doing that operation is no fun, you know."

"That seems like way too much for something that little!" she complained.

"Let me explain it then," I said. "The anesthesia is difficult because skunks are real sensitive. Then, the surgery is also delicate because the glands are located in a very sensitive and out-of-the-way place. If one of the thin-walled scent glands happens to get nicked during the surgery, then that terrible smell gets all over me and inside my surgical area. Then my wife and children won't have anything to do with me for weeks, nor will I have any clients to come into my place."

"But Dr. Jenkins said you could do it at his taxidermy shop. He won't mind if it gets a little smelly in there. It smells funny in there anyway."

"Well, OK," I said, giving in. "I'll do it for fifteen dollars each."

"Fine," she said, "I'll have all five of 'em at Carney Sam's shop first thing in the morning."

"Five! I didn't know you had that many!"

There are only a handful of so-called "skunk descenters" in the entire world, and most of them, including me, would prefer to remain anonymous. You will find medical specialists of all kinds listed in the Yellow Pages, including board-certified orthopedic surgeons, cardiologists, oncologists, veterinary dermatologists, and even feline behavioral specialists, but you'll never find anyone who publicly owns up to being a skunk descenter. It's not that they are ashamed of their work, it's just that they would just as soon never do another one.

Years ago, it was considered all right to descent skunks. Nowadays, the Veterinary Association suggests that people shouldn't keep skunks as pets since they have been known to carry the rabies virus. Therefore, they don't condone veterinarians performing the surgery.

But in 1963 the procedure was perfectly legal, for any vet fool enough to do it. So early the next morning I was sitting in my truck in front of Carney Sam's taxidermy shop, listening to sad country music songs and waiting patiently for the skunk lady. Carney Sam was nowhere to be seen. Since his old International truck was there, parked backward up on a large pile of red dirt, I assumed he was around somewhere, probably down at the barn feeding up his livestock or out at the dog pens fooling with his deer dogs.

A little while after daylight she rattled up in an old Dodge pickup, squealed to a stop, and quickly detrucked, holding a cardboard box out from her bosom as if it contained dynamite. Big letters on the side declared that the contents of the box were products of E. and J. Gallo. I noticed a faint but distinct skunk odor.

"I've brought these baby skunks and I wondered if I could leave 'em, then pick 'em up when I get off work over at the Vanity Fair plant."

"Yes ma'am, I'm sure Carney, er, Dr. Jenkins won't mind. Where did you find these babies?" I asked, opening up the wine box and peeking inside. They were little balls of white-and-black fur, crawling around ever so slowly like blind baby kittens, and they were making little chicklike sounds. Now the smell was getting intense.

"My husband ran over the momma with the tractor while he was hauling manure out of the hall of the barn. She and her babies were holed up in a pile of straw, and he couldn't tell they were there. He feels real bad about it so he's feeding them milk with a doll bottle every few hours. I tell you, Mr. McCormack, things don't smell too good around our place right now!"

After she left, I thought about how much trouble these folks were going to in order to save the little ones. Many people would have just walked away and forgotten them, primarily because of the disagreeable aroma. But these people understood that the smell was no fault of the babies, since they were too young to know about spraying their scent as a means of defense. I reckoned the odor in the box was left over from their recently departed mother.

I slowly retrieved my skunk surgical equipment from the truck, deliberately killing time until Carney Sam showed up. As I entered the taxidermy shop carrying skunks under one arm and medicine under the other, I heard his voice.

"Is that you, Doc? Has she gone?"

The voice came from over amongst a group of stuffed heads and whole body mounts. Deer heads were lying around, most upside down and pointing their antlers toward the ceiling, while a rigid bobcat in mid-hiss dared me to cross the imaginary line into his space. The scene also featured a beautiful red fox, several largemouth bass, and a red-tailed hawk in full wingspread, peering hungrily down at the uninvited stranger. The exhibition was impressive but eerie.

Suddenly, a red Funk's G Hybrid seed corn cap rose up. It was Carney.

"What're you doing, boy?" I asked.

"Is she gone?"

"Yeah, she's been gone!" I declared. "Why are you hiding?"

"Well Doc, I just didn't want her to know that I couldn't fix those skunks. 'Course I think I could, but I ain't got the medicine to put 'em to sleep with," he replied. "You know the govmunt keeps that dope stuff under tight control."

"Come on Carney, stop complaining about the government and let's get this skunk business over with," I suggested.

"Well, OK. But I want you to show me how it's done. 'Course I won't be able to do it, but I want to see it."

My method of skunk anesthesia in the 1960s would probably be frowned upon by veterinary anesthesiologists and malpractice lawyers today, even though it was a very safe, inexpensive, and practical dirt-road contraption. The anesthetizing chamber was a cardboard box that had once contained a gallon jug of bovine rumen tonic. The chamber was activated by placing an ether-saturated wad of cotton in the bottom of the box, introducing the skunk, and then quickly sealing the box shut with tape. As long as the patient was awake, he could be heard scratching around inside the chamber, but when he reached Stage One of surgical anesthesia, the scratching ceased. At that point, I would remove the patient and perform the surgery.

Shortly, I had one of the patients sealed in the anesthetic chamber and the ether was doing its job. A few minutes later, I was showing Carney the procedure.

"See here, Carney. You squeeze right here on the sides of his rear, and the tip of the scent gland pooches out a little. Now I grasp that with these forceps, then I take this scalpel and very carefully tease and dissect it out."

Our faces were less than a foot from the surgical area and the penetrating odor encouraged me to be quick about the job.

"If you aren't careful, you will make a mislick and then you've got a mess," I lectured.

The words had no more escaped my lips when I committed the grievous error of rupturing the sac. Green juice geysered wildly into the air, making a direct hit in Carney's right eye, setting his cornea on fire.

"*Aaaaghhhh!*" screamed Carney as he jumped back and started dancing around, clawing at his eye. "*I'm blind!*"

From previous experience, I knew that Carney was as tough as corncobs and gravel. About the only time he exhibited any hint of pain was when something happened to his eyes. He could get his feet stomped on by wild yearlings or his thighs kicked by undisciplined backyard plug horses and he would only flinch. But if trash blew in his eyes or if someone directed a flashlight beam in that direction, he would act like he had been jabbed with an electric cattle prod.

"Carney, quit scratching at your eye!" I yelled. "Get to the sink and get some water in it!"

While we were cupping faucet water with our hands and frantically sloshing it into his eye, I glanced back over to my patient. The little varmint was semiawake and crawling dangerously close to the edge of the table. One more step and he would nosedive onto the cold concrete below. I lunged toward the table and caught the beast just as he tumbled.

I redeposited my patient back into the skunk-anesthetizing chamber, poured more ether onto the cotton wad, and sealed the chamber shut with more tape. Then I went back to check on the condition of my associate.

Carney was opening and shutting his eye in testing fashion. Although it was red as a pinkeyed cow's, he claimed that the pain had subsided and that he could see almost as well as before the accident.

"Reckon you ought to go to the doctor," I asked, "or do you just want me to put some mastitis medicine in it?"

"Naw, it's OK I think," he replied. "I'll just squirt some bull penicillin in it tonight if it still looks red then."

I had been keeping my ears tuned in to the signaling device of the anesthetizing chamber and when the scratching ceased, I unsealed the box to find the little fellow sleeping soundly. With some difficulty, I finally half-teased and half-incised the remainder of the stubborn scent gland from its bed. The second gland came away nicely, which renewed my confidence in my surgical ability.

I quickly anesthetized the others all together and completed the surgery without incident and without Carney Sam. He apparently had urgent business outside the building. It was certainly understandable since the inside reeked of skunk scent. Together with the formaldehyde that Carney used in embalming his animals, the odor was burning my eyes, nose, and even my exposed skin. It was a relief to finally complete the task and exit the premises.

I stopped at the creek on the way home, stripped under the bridge, and washed down with germicidal soap. Even though I had some residual skunk odor on my person and in my trunk, it was minor compared to poor old Carney Sam. He went to the hospital that night for emergency eye treatment and his veterinary business fell off considerably for the next few weeks. Several people came to our house with their pets for treatment.

"We usually use Dr. Jenkins because he's cheap, but recently his place has been smelling so bad!" one lady declared, holding her overweight Pomeranian.

"Looks to me like the govmunt ought to step in and make some of these veterinarians clean up their acts," another outraged pet lover declared. "Dr. McCormack, you simply must report Dr. Jenkins to the authorities for having such a horrible facility in which he houses our beloved pets. We took our little dog Sweetums there for treatment and now poor Sweetums smells like a polecat. What can we do? We'll never go there again!"

I couldn't help but be amused at the reaction of the public. They didn't seem to mind taking their beloved pets to an unlicensed vet for treatment, but it was an outrage that his building was smelly. Of course, Carney could not divulge the source of the odor, nor could I. But I did vow to perform future skunk-descenting operations out in the pine woods and to always wear a rain suit.

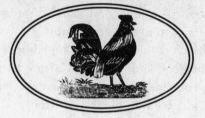

Chapter 22

THE LONG-DISTANCE call was from Picayune, a long way from Choctaw County.

"Doctuh," she announced, "this is Mrs. Toone from Picayune. My little Chihuahua, Tiguh, is quite ill and needs immediate medical attention. Can you see him right away?"

Certain words and phrases are red flags for veterinarians. The word "Chihuahua," or "the bank's on the phone," or "forty cows down" are signals that tell the astute veterinarian that trouble and stress are just ahead. Therefore, it is time to gird one's loins for a physical and psychological battle.

I don't think that Chihuahuas and other small lapdogs are mean, it's just that they are often spoiled and not properly disciplined by their indulgent owners. But if I had a choice between a two-thousand-pound Brahman bull or a Chihuahua, I'd take the bull.

"How long will it take you to get here?" I asked.

"Three and a half hours," she said, "unless I have cah trouble."

"Ma'am, don't you have a vet there? That sure is a long way to drive," I exclaimed.

"Yes, I know, Doctuh," she said smoothly, "but I've heard so much about how good you are with pets. You saved my sister's little dog. You remember her, Mrs. Merriman from Meridian and her little Pekingese, Ming Toy?"

Lordy, did I remember! That Peke wasn't a dog, it was a popeyed crocodile with its tail cut off! It took the whole community to treat the fool thing. Half to hold him, while the other half wrung their hemorrhaging hands in agony, after he had quickly and gleefully chomped on their unsuspecting fingertips.

"Oh yes, I do remember Ming Toy. I hope he's well and healthy," I said sweetly through clenched teeth.

"Yes, he's doing well, thanks to your wonderful skill and love of animals," she cooed. "None of the vets here seem to love animals like you do."

Young vets should not let such bragging go to their heads, especially when such flattery is issued by potential clients from distant towns where there is an ample supply of competent colleagues. The client may be well justified in raving about your great skill in saving the animal kingdom. On the other hand, it more likely could be that he or she owes overdue bills to the local practitioners, or there has been some run-in about the manners of the client's pet, or something of that nature.

I know all this now. That day, of course, I accepted the case and told Mrs. Toone that I would be waiting for her at the appointed hour.

About four hours later, the wealthy widow slowly eased her old black Buick Roadmaster into the driveway. I could see the tiny dog standing on the seat beside her with his front feet propped up on the dash. The lady immediately started reaching over to the passenger side and into the back seat, pulling together numerous quilts, blankets, and afghans. When she emerged from the car, Tiger was wrapped in no less than twenty-five pounds of woolen goods. On this unusually warm winter afternoon his mistress looked like a new mother taking a two-day-old infant home from a Siberian hospital in thirty-five-below-zero weather.

She entered my little clinic room with great authority, strode briskly to the examination table, and commenced slowly unwrapping the patient as if it were a fiftieth wedding anniversary gift. After several seconds of peeling off layer upon layer of blankets, there he sat.

"Hello, Tiger," I said slowly and softly, while carefully easing my hand toward the mass of blankets.

This careful attempt at friendship was greeted by a sudden springing to his feet, a vicious and snapping series of growl-barks, and the short hair on his back standing on end.

"Oh, don't hurt him, he's so sweet," sympathetically cried Mrs. Toone.

At that instant I would rather have been dehorning five hundred head of Brahman bulls in south Texas.

Let me try to describe Tiger. He was the typical overweight, sickly, five-year-old Chihuahua, weighing about six pounds. His numerous teeth, both deciduous and permanent, were all the color of half-rotten bananas. His breath had the odor of an eight-day-old retained cow placenta in late August. On the left side of his upper jaw was a draining tract from an abscessed upper fourth premolar. When he coughed and gagged up white saliva, I could see two huge and fiery-red tonsils the size of hulled walnuts protruding from their crypts. His attire consisted of a small red collar with a Christmas bell on it and a navy blue, obviously hand-knitted doggy sweater. His toenails were painted red and were adequately long for scaling stone mountains. Some of his claws had even grown completely around in a circle and were growing back into the flesh of his feet.

He exhibited a small remnant of an umbilical hernia and had a hairless area the size of a poplar tree leaf just behind his lumbar region. There was evidence of bilateral knee problems and cruciate ligament damage. His anal glands were the size of Ping-Pong balls. He was also blessed with tapeworms. Here was a perfect example of a pathologist's dream and a practitioner's nightmare.

"Why don't you tell me what seems to be troubling Tiger," I suggested, with hands tightly clasped behind my back.

"Why he's just a sick little fellow," she answered. "He's been coughing so much, then gags up foam. He has diarrhea a lot of the time, and he won't eat anything except canned chicken and baby food."

"Yes ma'am," I replied quietly, while trying to act in an understanding manner. I wanted to rub my chin but didn't, for fear any hand or eye movement would initiate another canine tantrum.

"And he eats grass when I let him outside. Why does he eat grass?"

"Because it's there," I wanted to say, but didn't. I felt like Mrs. Toone was not in any mood for frivolity.

"And does he, uh, lick his rear end?"

"Oh yes, yes, all the time!" she declared.

"Uh huh. And does he scoot around on his rear end on the carpet a lot?"

"Oh yes, yes, exactly!"

"I see," I answered. I desperately wanted to rub my chin as if in deep thought and turn my gaze toward the ceiling, but things were just going too well to make any sudden moves.

"Does he sometimes feel bad and cough a lot late at night?"

"Yes, you're exactly right. Oh, you know so much about little dogs! I'm so glad I finally found someone who likes small animals!" she gushed.

"Yes ma'am," I replied, deadpan. This time I forgot and my left hand involuntarily advanced upward. Before it even reached shoulder level, the atmosphere was pierced with a series of yap-growls so shrill and violent that it sent a chill up my spine. I'm sure I jumped as if suddenly struck with a cattle prod.

"Tiguh! Shame, shame on you! Don't snap at the wonderful doctor. He's just trying to help you. He loves you, too!"

I bit the inside of my lower lip and said nothing. I wanted to give her a lecture on discipline, but when you work with people, many things are better left unsaid. Right now I just wanted to get on with the job.

"Mrs. Toone, why don't you leave him with me for a hour or so, and I'll give him a good examination. Then when you come back he'll be treated and ready to go," I suggested. "My wife is real good with pets and she will assist me."

"Oh, I do hate to leave him, even for an hour, but I suppose I could if your wife will look after him. He does seem to like women a lot better than men."

"Sure enough! I thought it was my cologne!" I heard myself say. "Or maybe my kennel-side manner needs a little upgrading."

A wee smile graced her pursed lips. Perhaps she did have a sense of humor after all.

"This will be his private room right here," I declared, pointing to one of two cages at the end of the room. "I think he will find the accommodations here quiet and comfy." Another smile crossed her lips, just before she kissed his mishapen head and slipped him into his temporary quarters.

After she left, I peeked in on Tiger. He growled when my hand invaded his space, then barked, snapped, and showed me all his teeth.

Restraining vicious dogs is a major problem for veterinarians.

Medium- and large-size dogs can be muzzled, or in extreme cases, injected with a sedative or anesthetic. But small Chihuahuas and Pekes can't be handled like big dogs. They need to be blanketed.

"We've got a blanket case out here in a cage," I told Jan a few minutes later in the kitchen, "and I need your help with the sweet thing."

Back in my tiny clinic room, I retrieved my old green army blanket and a pair of heavy gloves from the top shelf.

When I tossed the blanket atop Tiger, he became a wiggling, writhing, and biting demon, but that helped in rolling him up in the blankety mass.

"Don't hurt him, John. Remember, he's not a bull!" Jan said as she pulled on the gloves. "You've got to learn to be more gentle with these little ones. They're so fragile."

"Don't worry, I'm being careful. The blanket is real soft and this method of restraint is approved by the AVMA. This way he can't hurt himself or somebody else." I wondered why I was spouting such drivel, but it did sound good.

"Yeah, right," she said sarcastically. "Save that line for somebody else."

Once the squirming ceased within the blanket, I began to peel off layers until the top of Tiger's head was visible. Then while my blood epinephrine level was still high, I grasped his neck right behind the ears and extracted him, snarling and slobbering, from the blanket. His mouth was gaped open, possum style, and his eyes were bulged out but were still shooting poison daggers at his new enemy.

"OK Jan, now get 'im!" I stated through gritted teeth.

Soon Jan held his head tightly cradled in her gloved hands and she was softly cooing all the correct and soothing phrases in her best little-dog voice. And it was working! Tiger calmed down due to her expertise in canine relations and perhaps because I was standing behind them and out of sight. But when I touched his behind, he became unglued again. Again, soothing words from Jan calmed his fears.

"Hang on, honey, I'm gonna work up from this end."

I quickly inserted a thermometer in his rear, then stethoscoped his chest, palpated his abdomen, and then clipped his toenails, all done with less difficulty than I imagined.

"Temperature of one-oh-four-point-five degrees! No wonder he's sick!" I told Jan.

Next, I took a wad of cotton and expressed a large quantity of fetid fluid from his anal glands.

"I *thought* he had inflamed anal glands! No wonder he's been scratching and scooting his hind end on her carpet," I said. "I'll bet his throat is as red as his rear. Let's take a tongue depressor and have a look."

I thought Tiger had calmed down enough for an oral exam, but I was dead wrong. When I stuck the little wooden paddle into his mouth he immediately chomped it in half and proceeded to crush his half into a thousand pieces before spitting out the saliva-saturated splinters. The look in his eyes told me he was very pleased with himself and he double-dog-dared me to stick anything else between his powerful jaws.

"Sure looks like a rip-roaring case of tonsillitis to me," I diagnosed. "Just look at the size of those lymph glands!"

"Yep, looks like it to me, too," Jan concurred.

Seconds later I was injecting his leg with penicillin, which caused another struggle complete with more writhing, yelling, and glaring. But then it was over, and he was back in his chamber, free of the restraints and probing of his tormentors.

When Mrs. Toone returned, I pointed out all of Tiger's numerous health problems. She, however, was only interested in his rear end and throat problems. She did agree to brush his teeth every day with salt and soda and give him a tapeworm treatment.

After her second visit, I suggested that she consider the possibility of a tonsillectomy for Tiger. The reaction I received was as if I had suggested he undergo a frontal lobotomy and leg amputation. She immediately grabbed Tiger, clutched him to her ample bosom, and showered him with kisses and nauseating sweet talk.

"He's all the family I have," she whispered with tears in her eyes. "He even sleeps in my bed on his own little pillow."

Eventually, though, the trips from Picayune became more frequent for "throat and gland" treatment. One weekend Mrs. Toone called and told me that she had finally decided to take my advice about the surgery.

"I'd like to bring him in early Monday morning," she requested, "and leave him with you the rest of the week."

This was an unusual request, since in all the previous visits she had never left Tiger alone in my presence for more than a couple of hours.

"I'm remarrying on Tuesday," she said coyly, "and I just know that you'll take good care of my baby. I'll be moving to Texas with my new husband within a month."

The tonsillectomy was routine, with no problems or complications. Tiger even acted like something other than the uncouth hellion that we had come to expect. When he realized that "his momma" wasn't there, he even ate Purina dry dog food and drank cold faucet water like a normal dog.

On Wednesday, Tiger's owner called while I was out and asked about him, but later Jan revealed that she wasn't her usual nervous self. She also was somewhat vague about when she would be by to pick him up and didn't even ask about his appetite. Could it be that Tiger had been demoted to second-class citizenship and the new husband was now occupying the position previously held by the little dog?

I was out doing herd work when the lady came by, picked Tiger up, and paid her bill. Jan said she paid the bill and almost forgot about the patient. She and her new husband drove off in a new pickup truck with a shocked Tiger standing all alone in a bird dog box in the back.

Sometime later, I met her while walking down the street. She had changed her hair, her clothes were different, and in general she just acted like a new person.

"Why Mrs. Toone, what are you doing in Butler?" I asked.

"Oh, I'm here visiting my sister. She just moved over here from Meridian. She got tired of the big city and decided to move to the country."

"I see." Certainly Meridian was a lot bigger than Butler, but I never thought of it as a "big city." "Well, how are you doing, Mrs. Toone?"

"Just fine, Doctuh," she cooed, "but I'm now Mrs. Brown from Baytown. My husband is a roughneck who works in the oil field."

"Well, it's obvious that you are very happy," I offered, "but tell me, how's Tiger?"

"Who? Tiguh?" she asked, puzzled. "Oh, Tiguh! Oh, he's fine. Haven't had a minute's trouble with that throat or those glands since. He's an outside dog now. Plays with Mr. Brown's bird dogs all the time. The surgery made a new dog out of him."

"Well, I declare!" I exclaimed. That verified what I had always thought. Once a spoiled lapdog is treated like a regular dog, it gets the message that improper behavior is a liability.

Every human needs something or somebody to love, and frequently it is an animal of some kind. In many cases the human/animal bond is stronger and holds more love than human/human relationships. Of course, even a pet ought to be mannerly, whether at home or on the road, since there may be someone out there just waiting to take its place. He or she might wake up one morning with a sore throat and rear end, but have no soft pillow or bed to lay them on.

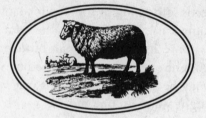

Chapter 23

"How come calves don't eat french fries?"

"Why don't horses wear clothes?"

"How does a cat purr?"

Tom, our oldest child, could always ask the most thought-provoking questions and ask them faster than any little boy I've ever seen.

Busy veterinarians don't get to see their children as much as they would like. Too often they leave home before the kids awaken, then get home after they are in bed asleep. One solution to that problem is to take them along on calls occasionally. This also allows mommas to have a little time for themselves.

Tom went with me on his first large animal call when I was interning with Dr. Foreman in Baldwin County. He was about a year old, more or less, when I drove the truck right up to the corral fence so that he and Jan would have ringside seats to observe the birth of a calf. When the happy event resulted in two live calves instead of only one, he clapped his hands with glee. His excitement was matched by that of his mother, father, and the owner of the cow.

A few months later, he held a bottle of calcium at just the right height when we were treating a milk fever case at John Dillon's dairy. Can you imagine trying to explain to a two-year-old exactly why a big, beautiful black-and-white cow is down, comatose, and can't get up? It's similar to the time I attempted to define the duties of a farm veterinarian, in understandable terms, to a cab driver in the big city. I found that both are a challenge to your communication skills.

Our most memorable call together came when a typical calving problem was phoned in about seven P.M. one unexpectedly pleasant winter evening. Tommy was about four at that time.

"Daddy, may I go with you, please?" he asked.

"Ask your momma," I replied, as I hung up the phone.

Jan was not particularly pleased with the idea because of the lateness of the hour, but she agreed anyway since Tommy truly wanted to observe his second obstetrical procedure.

"Now don't get dirty, or too cold, and watch out where you step," she ordered, "and y'all get home before nine."

"I'm sure we won't be too long," I reckoned. "It probably will be just a simple delivery."

The possibility of a long, drawn-out birthing did cross my mind, as did a cesarian section, but I figured that the odds for a quick job and a speedy return home were in my favor.

The eighteen-mile country road trip was especially enjoyable since Tom's conversation covered many subjects along the way. He asked about many species of animals, questioned me closely about the use of silos, and fired numerous other questions at me.

Upon arrival at the farm, we discovered that the heifer in question was not corralled, but was running free in the orchard.

"She's down, Doc," the farmer replied. "We'll just drive right up to her and drop the rope over her head. She's not in any shape to cause us any trouble."

I knew those words were a warning signal, but this time I thought we were going to be lucky. We slowly drove the truck right up to the fence about fifty feet from where the laboring heifer was lying, and she didn't attempt to hop up and run off. However, as we got out and approached her from the rear, she rose energetically and started to sprint away from the intruders.

Now, some of my veterinary colleagues allow as how they never have to rope or "cowboy" any of their patients. According to what they tell me, they wouldn't waste their time doing that kind of nonveterinary task even if the cow was owned by an elderly, invalid, shut-in lady who had no corral or barn. I do not understand how they get their patients treated.

I have found that it is often more expedient to go ahead and make an effort to catch the cow than it is to leave, return later, and make a second trip charge.

When we were in veterinary school, my colleagues and I all possessed nice nylon lariats, and we practiced throwing them on garbage cans, fence posts, one another, or any other ropable object nearby. We knew that we would, of necessity, need some degree of roping skill when we started our practices.

As the heifer started to move away from us, I sprinted out to flank her proposed escape route, twirled the lariat over my head a couple of times, and let it fly. The garbage-can practice had paid off again! When the loop fell cleanly over her head, I trotted along with her to the next apple tree, around which I made a quick loop. Two seconds later the heifer was stopped abruptly when she reached the end of her rope.

When I glanced back at the truck, I could see Tom standing on the seat, looking out the window, and clapping his hands excitedly. I suppose he had seen enough Western TV shows to know that catching a bucking bovine with a rope was good and deserved applause.

After we had the patient restrained, I pulled the truck up close and directed the beam of the headlights into the working area. While I made my examination, Tom crawled out the truck window and sat on the hood, watching every move the cow and I both made.

"I thought you were gonna stay in the truck, hoss," I said.

"I can't see, Daddy. May I stay here?" he asked.

By then I had decided that a cesarian section was the best alternative for the poor beast. The fetus was oversized and the heifer's pelvic opening was too small. I injected a tranquilizer, dropped her on the ground, and tied up her legs. I was shaving and scrubbing the incision site when Tom spoke up again.

"Daddy, I gotta go to the bathroom!" he blurted out.

His bold announcement froze my soapy hands in midair. The farmer and his farmhands snickered and exchanged glances in amusement as I dried my hands and went to give assistance.

When we returned, I grabbed a plastic bucket and turned it upside down right next to where I would be doing the surgery.

"Now Tom," I ordered, "you sit right here on this bucket and watch what I do, so you can do it next time."

For the next few minutes, he watched what I was doing very closely. Although this was his first C-section, he had observed other surgeries on small animals, so he knew enough about surgical technique to converse about it.

"There's a bleeder, Daddy," he advised as my incision extended into muscle and cut through an artery.

"The cow's eyes are open, Daddy."

"Can't you find the calf, Daddy?" he asked as I buried both hands and arms inside the cow's belly and struggled in an attempt to bring the calf to the outside.

"Shhh, shhh!" I said. "Don't talk so much. I've got to think!"

After that advisement, I could hear him whispering quietly to himself and squirming on the bucket.

Suddenly the calf popped through the incision and the two farmhands pulled him off to the side.

"Tom, get one of those towels and rub him real hard," I ordered. "Rub hard!"

"He's wet and slippery," Tom said, "and he's shaking his head!"

"That's good! Keep on rubbing him!"

As I closed the incision, one of the hands pulled another truck up close and turned on the lights. "It's amazing how much easier suturing is when you can see," I declared.

"That's good," Tom said. "I can see better now myself." Apparently he thought the lights were arranged for his benefit.

"You getting sleepy, hoss?" I asked.

"No sir!" he replied with vigor.

Soon the little calf was sitting up, snorting and shaking his head. Tom was chatting with him as he continued the rubdown. Every few minutes he would look over my shoulder.

"Whatcha doin' now, Daddy?" he asked several times.

"Aw, I'm trying to get her sewed up. We're almost through."

Finally we finished, got the heifer to her feet, and she was introduced to her new baby. As we got into the truck and left, the calf was trying to find the proper spot to nurse and its mother was sniffing and licking her new offspring.

By the time we got down the long driveway and onto the county road, Tom began to lie down in the seat. It was past his bedtime and he was exhausted from his exciting evening activity.

As he eased down in the seat beside me following a big yawn, he said, "Daddy, how old do I have to be to operate on a momma cow and find a baby?"

"You'll have to study hard as you're growing up and then go to a special school to learn how," I answered.

He thought about that as his eyelids drooped and he said, "Daddy, I bet you're the bestest doctor in the whole world."

I thought about that as I drove home. When I looked down into that beautiful sleeping face I certainly didn't believe I was the bestest doctor in the whole world, but I knew for certain that I was the luckiest daddy in the whole world.

"Where have y'all been?" Jan exclaimed when I walked into the house with Tom asleep on my shoulder. "I've been worried sick! I just knew you had been in an accident. This child should have been in bed long ago! And just look at those shoes. They're filthy and smelly!"

We immediately put him to bed, only taking time to remove his shoes and socks. There was no need of awakening him to put on pajamas. I told Jan all about the events of the past couple of hours as we stood there beside his bed holding hands for a few minutes. I wondered if he would long remember the event that he had just witnessed. Someday would he look back and recollect the miracle of birth and the way he stimulated the little calf to breathe?

Some twenty years later I asked Tom if he remembered the incident.

"No sir, not that specific one," he replied. "But I do remember other similar episodes. The main thing I remember is that you always had to rope the cow and it was usually at night."

That's the same memory I have of most of those calls. But when the children were along, events were a lot more interesting.

I wish it were possible for all children to have a little exposure to agriculture. It would teach them a lot of biology, as well as show them that their milk, meat, fruit, and vegetables do not magically appear from the back room of the supermarket. If they could see how much effort goes into getting a hamburger and a tomato into the kitchen, they would have a better appreciation for those who supply our food.

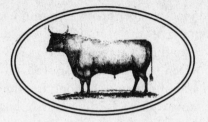

Chapter 24

IT WAS A rainy Friday evening in February and I was watching late-night TV in the company of a newly acquired and scrawny-looking kitten. Tom and Lisa were having a difficult time selecting a suitable name for the gray tabby, although several possibilities had been suggested. Tom thought the name "Fred" would be nice, while Lisa suggested "Kitty," and then Jan diplomatically suggested that neither name was quite original enough for such a scruffy specimen of feline flesh. I thought "Worms" might be appropriate.

Jan wanted a name with a Southern flavor. She had mentioned J.D., which was short for Jefferson Davis, then George, Bubba, Buck, Bear, and Shug. All good Southern names, which represented political figures or famous football coaches. All except Bubba and Buck, of course, and those handles would make any good cat proud to be a product of the South.

Our TV fare was an episode of *Combat,* my favorite series. An American tank blasted through a rock wall and the GIs were following it through the gap. No doubt victory was imminent! Suddenly, amongst the crackle of M-1 rifle fire and whistling incoming missiles, our dog Mickey started to bark one of those somebody's-out-here barks out on the porch. Presently I heard several sharp raps on the screen door.

"Who could that be," I said to myself, depositing the cat on the couch, "out here in this rain and so late at night?" I quickly barefooted it to the door, snapped on the porch light, and opened the door.

"I'm looking for the veterinary," the visitor said. It was Benny Lee, Rufus Campbell's hired man. He was attired in an old cowboy hat, yellow poncho, and black rubber boots. The rain had soaked through his hat and was dripping off the brim, which was turned down all the way around. He was holding a kerosene lantern in one hand.

Benny Lee was much of a man, his six-feet-four figure carrying some two hundred and fifty pounds of bone and double muscle seemingly cut from the same pattern as Mule Marsh, boar hog owner and field hand of Mr. Kent Farris. I suppose today Benny's proper title would be "agricultural commodity aide," or something equally asinine. Benny Lee was the "main man," or "farm land associate," of Mr. Rufus Campbell, an important landholder, cattleman, and sawmill operator in the eastern part of the county.

I had seen Benny Lee once before at the feed store, where he was tossing hundred-pound sacks of grain around with one hand while the regular store sitters urged him on. A little later he was picking up an anvil with one hand and doing one-handed chin-ups on the exposed ceiling joists.

"I'm the veterinarian," I said. "What can I do for you?" The Southern spring rain was beating a tattoo on the porch roof, as the thunder rolled and lightning flashed.

"Mr. Campbell, he sent me to git you, Doc," he answered. "The telephone's out, on account of all this here rain."

"OK, what's wrong, Benny Lee?"

"Uh, Mr. Campbell, he said for me to tell you that one of his hosses has cut hisself real bad and he's bleedin' somethin' fierce," he declared. I noticed he wasn't looking me in the eye, and at the time I wondered why. It worries me when livestock folks won't look me in the eye.

"OK, let me get my boots on and I'll be right on, or if you want to wait, I'll just follow you out to the barn."

"Well, uh, he ain't at the barn," he said kind of slowlike.

Large animal vets quickly learn to pick up certain signals from the way things are said, as well as from what is said, or sometimes not said. Statements that begin with "Uh, well" or "He's just a plum pet, Doc" or "We'll have her caught up by the time you get here" are surefire verbal indications that a long and difficult call is ahead.

"Where is he?" I asked, reaching for my boots.

"Uh, well, he's across the Tombigbee River in the Marengo Swamp. Mr. Campbell, he's got a boat down there that we can go across in," he said proudly.

I was reaching for my boots but stopped in midgrab.

"You mean we've got to go across that river with it out of banks and that current so swift!" I stammered, with my jaw dropped.

"Yessuh, that's right."

Two of the things that I fear the most are high places and high water! I have nightmares of falling off tall silos in West Virginia and drowning while trying to swim across the flood-swollen Elk River. The Tombigbee River was only a hundred yards wide normally, but I knew that it would be much wider that night since it was flooded out into the river bottoms.

"Can't we go up and cross at the bridge?" I pleaded weakly.

"Uh, well, we could, but that would be about a thirty-mile trip. If we cross at Mount Sterling, it'll only be eight from right here," he explained.

I knew there was no point in further negotiation, so I slipped on my boots, rustled into a raincoat, grabbed an extra flashlight, and scribbled a note for Jan, just in case. Then I plunged out the door and into the rain.

Seconds later I was in my truck, following Benny Lee out the driveway and down the road. By then the almost constant rain of the past few days had slowed to a drizzle, but there were still huge puddles of water all along the road. In some areas the ditches had overflowed, resulting in sheets of water cascading across the pavement. Chunks of wood, tree limbs, and debris littered the roadway.

When the paved road ran out, we cautiously felt our way along the clay-based road, which was now a mushy twenty-foot-wide strip of red mud and water. Since I was following Benny Lee, I kept a safe distance from his rear wheels in order to maintain a semiclean windshield. The old truck in front of me frequently fishtailed and sashayed around when its wheels ran out of the watery ruts created by previous vehicles.

As we neared the river, the late-night fog suddenly became much thicker, which created a visibility problem. I continued following the old truck closely, my eyes glued to the glow of its taillights. Suddenly, the truck's brake lights came on and it made a hard left turn down a short ramp.

"Doc, let's put all yo' stuff in this boat here," Benny Lee ordered. "The hoss is downstream 'bout half a mile."

As I peered anxiously at the ten-foot johnboat, we loaded it up with my two black bags, rope, instruments, bucket, and flashlight. I didn't think we'd need to take a jug of water because we were surrounded with a plenteous supply.

We then waded out into the water, and shakily stepped over into the boat.

"Don't turn us over, Doc," Benny Lee cried, as he held on to the sides.

"I don't like this a little bit!" I yelled. "We're gonna get out in this river and capsize!" I started untying my boots. If we had to swim, I reckoned that I'd at least have light feet!

Benny Lee quickly inserted a wad of Red Man into his right cheek and commenced jerking on the rope to the old Johnson motor. After several yanks it started sputtering, and we were soon cautiously making our way out between the flooded trees.

Once out in the main channel, Benny turned right and steered downstream. Meanwhile I sat frozen in the bow, one hand gripped on to the boat side, the other holding the flashlight aloft, trying to see through the foggy mist.

The beam emitted by the flashlight did little good, but it was better than nothing for identifying floating chunks and logs that we occasionally encountered. I tried to indicate the proper direction by using hand signs.

Whomp!

I jumped about six inches off the cold seat and quickly turned and fired a panicky glance at Benny Lee.

"Just a log, Doc. Didn't you see it?" he yelled above the huge noise of the little motor.

I shook my head and peered earnestly into the murky waters. Shortly, I noticed that we were cutting across the flow. I reckoned that we must have been on about the same latitude as our patient. As the old motor labored to cut across the current, I searched the foggy darkness with my flashlight for obstructions. After a couple of minutes, the trees of the opposite bank appeared before my light and I started to breathe a little more freely. We eased between tree branches and slid to a stop in the gooey mud of the slough.

The steady drizzle on the trees was a welcome sound to my ears after the anxious droning of the outboard motor the past few minutes.

When I stood up and started collecting equipment, I realized that my knees were quivering like Jell-O. I tried hard to hide it because I didn't want Benny Lee telling everybody in the county about how scared Doc was of a little water.

With Benny Lee in front, we trudged quietly through a grove of cypress trees. Apparently neither of us was interested in initiating conversation. The two big bags, ropes, and other equipment hadn't been too heavy for the first two hundred yards or so, but now I was feeling the weight. The mud was making the trip unpleasant.

"How much farther?" I puffed.

"Not far, I reckon," he replied, peering anxiously through the fog. I wondered if he really knew where he was going.

A few minutes later, a high spot of ground appeared. It seemed to be a manmade mound some ten feet high, perhaps a hundred feet long and fifty feet wide. On top of the mound was a pole barn containing baled hay and a couple of enclosures. I assumed this was "high ground," where livestock could go when the river bottom flooded.

Inside one of the enclosures lay a yearling horse. As we approached the gate, he stood and looked at us timidly, shivering and shaking. Then I noticed the blood on his hind legs and as the beam of my light traveled upward, my jaw dropped at the sight I saw. At least three feet of something was loosely hanging from his groin.

"What in the world? What happened? Did he get crossways on a stump or something?" I stammered.

"Mr. Doc, I got to tell you the truth," Benny said slowly. "Mr. Campbell, he got Mr. Carney Sam to come out this morning to castrate this hoss. Then tonight when I came over here to check on the cows, I found him like this. Mr. Campbell said not to tell you Mr. Carney Sam had been heah, 'cause he didn't think you'd come if you knowed that."

One of the worst things that can happen to a horse or veterinarian is for the patient to herniate after a castration. Through no fault of the surgeon, once in a while the horse's intestines get into the inguinal canal after the surgery, and then they prolapse out the newly made incision. Once this occurs, the horse usually dies of shock unless quick action is taken and the viscera cleaned and stuffed back into the abdominal cavity. Massive amounts of fluid therapy and antibiotics are indicated.

"Poor old horse. And poor old Carney," I thought to myself. "If he knew I was out here in this terrible weather dealing with one of his cases, he'd be upset. He would want to be here working with me. It wasn't his fault that the horse herniated."

"Where's Mr. Campbell?" I asked.

"He's over to the country club this evenin', I believe," Benny Lee said, never looking my way.

"Well Benny, we've got ourselves in a real mess. I guess we'll have to destroy him 'cause there's very little chance for him to survive with all that stuff hanging out of his body."

"Oh no suh! Mr. Campbell, he paid a pile of money for this hoss. Got him out of Texas or Oklahoma. He wants you to do whatever you can to fix him up, and said to tell you not to worry 'bout the money."

"Oh sure, I've heard that before!" I thought, but didn't say it. "Money's no object, because I probably won't get any of it whether he lives or dies." I was just a little peeved just thinking about Mr. Campbell over at the country club, eating steak and ice cream, and probably lighting five-dollar cigars with ten-dollar bills, while Benny Lee and I were struggling with a dying horse.

"Well, I don't think the horse has a chance to survive, but if that's what the man wants, that's what we'll do."

"Yessuh, he wants this little hoss to live," Benny declared.

I asked, "Got any clean water, Benny?"

"Yessuh. Got a well right over yonder." I was worried that muddy river water would not be good for cleaning live horse intestines.

While Benny went for water, I retrieved a bottle of seven percent chloral hydrate from my bag. I would have to get the horse anesthetized, up on his back, and his legs pulled forward. Chloral hydrate was not an especially good drug for a horse in shock, but it was all I had in my bag.

When Benny returned, I had everything ready and all my instruments draped out on a bale of hay just outside the stall. Once I got the horse down, I would bring the bale near the patient.

"You ever operate on a horse, Benny Lee?" I asked, hanging the lantern from a rafter.

"No suh! But I watched Mr. Carney Sam this afternoon when he worked on this 'un."

"Well, it's just me and you and this horse, and he's gonna be asleep.

So you'll have to be my assistant, hold this flashlight and hand me stuff."

In the eerie glow of the kerosene lantern light, I could see his gaze zeroing in on the shiny, mysterious implements, his eyelids so widely dilated that I could see a good half-inch of pearly eye white around the periphery of each dark brown iris.

"Yes suh!" he declared. "I'll he'p!"

Presently, I was holding the pint bottle aloft, watching the chloral disappear down the tube and through the sixteen-gauge needle into the patient's left jugular vein. I kept thinking about the narrow margin of anesthetic safety afforded by the drug and how deep the plane of anesthesia would have to be for me to get all the viscera returned to the horse's abdomen.

A couple of minutes later the horse's knees buckled and he started to weave and wobble.

"Just ease his head on down to the ground, Benny. Then hold on to him so he won't flop around," I said. After watching the way my assistant pinned the horse to the ground, patted its neck, and mumbled some easy words, I realized that as important as chemicals were, muscle power was still very useful for people who deal with equines.

I continued the IV for a few minutes more, slowing the flow by pinching the tube, until the patient reached what I estimated was light surgical anesthesia. There was no electrocardiogram, no blood pressure–measuring apparatus, and no anesthetic assistants, so I used the "look, listen, and feel" method of equine anesthesia.

This commonsense approach to anesthesia does not enjoy the popularity today that it did in the 1960s. Many horse owners have had abdominal surgery themselves and they would not want to be wrestled to the operating table by a Benny Lee. Therefore, they expect more sophisticated anesthetic techniques for their valuable equine companions. Cattle, however, are considered property by their owners and aren't usually afforded refined anesthetic techniques unless they are of high dollar value.

After we rolled the patient onto his back, we placed bales of hay on each side, which kept him from rolling from side to side. Then I began the scrub-down with water and disinfectant soap. To my surprise, most of the herniated mass was mesentery, which is the thin, sheetlike structure from which the intestines are suspended. There was a short intestinal loop protruding through the castration site some twelve to eighteen inches long, but luckily it seemed to be a normal pink-gray color. However, closer observation revealed a jagged laceration on the underneath portion. That portion of gut would have to be removed.

"Wash your hands real good, Benny. You're gonna have to help hold and stuff while I suture. But first, I've got to find another bucket."

While he scrubbed, I found an old zinc pail, the kind with a built-in nipple for feeding orphan calves. I filled it with water and poured in a few ounces of an iodine-based disinfectant. I would use that in place of sterile saline solution since there was none available. Next, I removed more instruments and suture material from the black bag and laid it with the other material on the towel atop the bale of hay. I quickly scrubbed again and in minutes was over the surgical site with instruments poised.

"We'll put a clamp here, and then another one here," I explained slowly, "because this piece of gut is torn and is almost gangrenous," I told Benny. "Then we'll remove it and sew the two ends back together." It's certainly easier to talk about than to do, especially on your knees in weak light.

But the sutures went in nicely, partly because Benny seemed to have a knack for holding the gut at just the right angle, which freed me up from trying to suture in all sorts of contorted angles. In minutes, suturing was complete, I tested for leaks, and the mesentery was closed.

"Now comes the hard part, Doctor," I told Benny. "We've got to get all this stuff back in the hole it came out of without doing any more damage to it."

"I don't know if it'll go back in that way," he stated, shaking his head.

"You start pouring a little of that water on it while I try to ease it back in."

I could feel the abdominal opening with my left hand and it was considerably bigger than it should have been. No doubt it was a congenital condition and herniation was inevitable, regardless of the surgeon. I made a mental note to remember to do a good physical in the future when I was called to castrate a horse.

Little things make vets happy. Things like observing a vigorous newborn lamb, or farmers who wave wildly when you meet them on the road, or prolapses that easily go back inside an animal like they are supposed to. I'm sure that things like this might puzzle regular citizens who've never been faced with such strange animal health problems.

With a minimum of grunting, groaning, and stuffing, the gut and mesentery finally slid back into the body cavity. I then blindly placed several heavy catgut sutures in the ring, placed a large pack of antibiotic-saturated cotton in the scrotum, and loosely sutured the skin closed. The patient had flinched several times when my needle pierced the body wall, so the anesthesia was beginning to wear off, just as I had wanted.

"What do you think, Benny?" I asked, carefully trying to get upright. I had begun to understand why large animal vets were such fast surgeons. It was because they performed so much of their surgery on their knees and bent over. If they stayed in that position too long, it took a long time to get sore knees and stiff backs into a standing position. The speedier the surgery, the easier it was on the musculoskeletal system of both man and beast.

I had begun to pick up instruments when I realized that Benny Lee had not answered my question. Perhaps he was thinking, or maybe he had not heard me. But then I realized he was mumbling. He was still on his knees, with head down and his hand placed on the patient.

"Lord, please heal dis hoss," he quietly pleaded, "if it's yo' will and you think best." He continued on about how much both he and Mr. Campbell thought of the horse and how difficult it would be to replace him. When he started to praise the Lord for this doctor who'd come out in the middle of the rainy night, I went to my knees too.

I had said prayers for sick animals before, but they had always been quick, quiet, and in the privacy of my own vehicle. But I'd never before found myself kneeling beside a horse and a praying man with my hand on his shoulder. While he prayed, I found myself wondering if prayer was mentioned anywhere in the veterinary literature. Then I wondered what my old hard-nosed, unsmiling professors would have thought, had they been on the scene. I didn't care, if it helped.

"Thank you for that kind prayer, Benny Lee. That's real nice of you," I said, when he was through. "You think the Lord will help us?"

"Well suh, I don't know for sure. But I do know that prayin' never hurt nobody."

"We've still got to give him a few shots," I replied, removing penicillin, cortisone, and two jugs of fluid from one of my bags. The two liters of fluid were only a fraction of the amount the dehydrated horse needed, but it was all I had.

Minutes later fluid was again bubbling through the rubber IV set into the patient's jugular vein. The flow of the precious fluid sounded as if it had a life of its own, the rhythmic glug-glugging mimicking the beating of a small heart.

Two liters of fluid, two syringes of penicillin, and a large dose of cortisone later, we managed to get the patient up in horse-sitting position. He was still groggy but was opening and shutting his eyes and trying to move his tongue around. After Benny Lee propped him up with two bales of hay, we stood back and looked.

It occurred to me that if this had been a television program and this horse had been a human patient in a people hospital, this would be the point in the crisis where the doctor would emerge from the sterile operating suite attired in his immaculate green scrub garb to talk to the apprehensive family.

"Well, it was touch-and-go there for a while, but he's going to be all right."

The family quickly and tearfully embrace, then the mother grasps the doctor's hand with both of hers.

"Thank you, Doctor. I'm so grateful for what you've done," she exclaims, tearfully pumping his hand appreciatively.

The doctor turns and walks back through the automatic doors of the OR, bathed in a glowing white light. The picture fades away, but the screen is blank for only a second; time for a Cadillac commercial.

As I looked down at my own attire, I had to smile. My wet coveralls were covered with blood, straw, and other foreign matter that defied description. My associate was likewise befouled. The only glow we emitted was the noxious aroma of an old stable mingled with the sick scent of a near-death equine.

"Think he's gonna make it, Benny?"

"It's all up to the Lord now," he said softly. "You done all you can do."

"I hope you're right," I replied.

We spent the next fifteen minutes or so washing up, cleaning instruments, gathering trash, and getting things packed back into their correct positions. Benny opened a new bale of hay and scattered it around the stall.

"You wanna go now, Doc, or what?" he asked.

"No, why don't we hang around awhile and see if we can get him standing in a little while. I think I'll lie down over there on those bales of hay."

Apparently I dozed off for a few minutes, because I was jolted awake by a commotion. I sat upright in time to see our patient standing on shaky legs, with Benny Lee steadying his head. While I watched, the horse took a couple of weak steps, then shook himself.

"Well that's a good sign," I said to myself. "If he can shake, he must not be near death."

Later he drank a few sips of water and lipped at some hay that Benny had offered. I was very pleased at his early progress, but realistically I knew that the odds were heavily stacked against his recovery.

"Let's go, Benny. We've done all we can do tonight." I gave the horse one last pat on the neck and off we trudged through the mud and mist.

When we arrived at boatside, I started untying my bootlaces, just as before.

"Whatcha doin' that for, Doc?"

"Aw, just in case we have a wreck in midstream and turn this thing over. You can't ever tell, we might get hit by a barge or get lost. I'll bet that water's deep!"

"Doc, let me tell you something," Benny said. "I've been running this river all my life and I know every trick she has. I know as much about this river as you know about doctoring on horses."

As we crossed the foggy river, I felt more confident than I had on the previous trip. I still kept my bootlaces loose, though, and kept a close watch for logs floating downstream. And I did close my eyes and utter a small prayer.

We soon arrived safely at the exact spot from where we had departed only a couple of hours before. It is still a mystery to me how Benny Lee piloted the boat so perfectly that foggy night, and why that horse survived.

Equines that herniate after castration, especially in dirty stalls, are not supposed to live. Even under the best of conditions, with sterile equipment, skilled assistance, and gallons of intravenous fluids, such cases are frequently lost.

I do not know whether Benny Lee and I received some help from a Higher Authority. It certainly wasn't because of any help we received from the country-clubbing Mr. Campbell and his pals. But that was just fine with me, because I followed my policy of adjusting the bill accordingly.

Today, every time I cross the bridge upstream over the Tombigbee River, I think about that rainy night with Benny Lee. I remember how panic-stricken I was crossing that swollen stream, and how much better I felt on my way back over after my cowboy navigator explained his qualifications to me. Nevertheless, every time I see deep water I still have a strong urge to pull my boots off and pray.

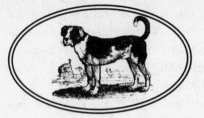

Chapter 25

AT ONE TIME, many general farmers possessed small sheep flocks. Lambs and wool provided a good source of income at a time of the year when most other crops were weeks or months away from harvest. However, as mutton consumption decreased and polyester fibers replaced wool, the ovine population dwindled, except in a few areas.

Although very few farmers own sheep in the Southeast, there are a considerable number of nonfarmers who have a few of them around just so they can watch the wooly creatures graze while proudly peering out the kitchen window. It makes them feel kind of "ag-like" and it also gives them an excuse to own a nice pickup truck.

Then there are the 4-H kids who work with a lamb or two as a project, often because they can't have a steer or heifer on the small space available. Feeding and showing a lamb is a great experience for a youngster.

Some sheep are kept just for their wool, so the lady of the house can spin it and make it into expensive sweaters. Regardless of who owns the sheep, once they cease to be raised solely for the purpose of meat, wool, or breeding stock, they become companion animals.

I have found that companion-animal owners expect and frequently demand the best in care for those animals. They expect their veterinarian to provide expert medical attention and care, often beyond the realm of common sense and economic value.

"You ought to just knock him in the head," Carney Sam Jenkins, my brusque, no-nonsense colleague, announced one afternoon to the wealthy owner of a wether named Sir Alfred. Sir Alfred was suffering from a blockage of his urinary tract, a common but serious affliction of male sheep, especially those that have been neutered. The very demanding owner, Mrs. Vanlandingham, quickly flew hot and requested that my colleague kindly remove himself from her estate in great haste. He gladly obliged since he didn't understand sheep health problems, nor did he care to acquaint himself with their unique characteristics. Sheep may be small ruminants, but they definitely are not small cows!

Mrs. Vanlandingham obtained my phone number from a sheep-lover colleague who had heard me lecture on sheep diseases to the FFA boys. She had been told that I owned a flock of sheep and it had also been rumored that I had actually healed a sheep once with my gifted hands.

It was true that I had once owned sheep. I had two of them, a ewe named Ziggy, who was too smart for her own good, and a ram named Bull-of-the-Woods. His name nicely revealed his personality.

The part about my actually "healing" a sheep by the laying on of hands was probably exaggerated. What really happened was that I saw a sheep hung up in a woven wire fence one day while driving down the gravel road. Naturally, I stopped and helped her out of her predicament.

To be perfectly truthful, it wasn't a sheep at all that was hung, it was a nanny goat. The only reason anybody even knew about it was because Goat the mailman passed by and observed me doing my daily good deed. And in spite of his name, Goat didn't know a goat from a sheep. He did like to talk, however; he was a great source of information and gossip in the county, second only to the barbershop. It wasn't long before folks like Mrs. Vanlandingham heard of my sheep skills.

When I arrived at the Vanlandingham estate, I found the very proper lady out in front of the mansion giving explicit orders to her team of submissive gardeners. As I got out of my truck, she dismissed the men with a couple of waves of her bejeweled hands. She was garnished with so many diamond rings and bracelets that she literally twinkled in the sunlight as she strode, queenlike, in my direction.

"I'll bet if she was touched by a strange human hand, sparks would fly," I grinned to myself, as I dusted off my coveralls and stood almost at attention.

Actually, I usually dislike working for rich people, entertainment stars, and big shots. They frequently are very demanding and want to give me orders about what I am to do and not to do with their animals.

"You must be the sheep specialist," she announced when she approached horseshoe-pitching distance from me and my truck. She wasn't smiling.

"Well, I'm no expert on sheep, but I do like them," I answered, trying to grin.

"Very well," she retorted, still stone-faced. "The patient is in the horse barn, in the last stall on the right. Please follow me."

I did as I was told, and within seconds we were entering a huge barn worth more than most houses that I had seen. All the stalls appeared to be vacant until we approached the end of the hallway. Suddenly, the bleat of a sheep came from the last one. Peering down over the partition, I saw an obese ovine standing amongst clean straw and several expensive blankets, peering back up at me.

"His name is Sir Alfred," she announced.

"How nice. Was he named after Alfred down at the feed store?" I asked.

"Of course not! He was named after one of my distant relatives in England," she declared, haughtily.

"Well, la-tee-da!" I thought to myself. "That probably explains another reason why Carney Sam was ejected from the premises. He probably didn't show sufficient respect for the ovine's alleged blue-blooded ancestry."

I decided not to ask anything more about the name, but instead made a complimentary comment regarding the situation.

"I see you have plenty of cover in there for him in case he gets cold. Good thinking! Most people wouldn't think of that, but you can't ever tell when a sick sheep might get a chill and need an extra blanket."

I couldn't believe I was actually saying such stuff out loud! And it sounded so convincing to my own ears, I was sure that she would think that I knew my business. Right away, her demeanor changed from arrogance to cool acceptance.

In short order I was examining the chunky ovine, checking eyes, ears, teeth, gums, feet, joints, and wool quality before using my stethoscope. All the time, the lady was reciting his ancestry, culinary preferences, and daily traffic patterns. While I stethoscoped his chest, her commentary continued, and I acknowledged her pronouncements by various head nods, eyebrow raises, and lip twitches.

I purposely delayed examination of his primary problem until I had looked at all other body systems. I was trying, through my examination procedure, to convince Mrs. Vanlandingham that I knew what I was doing, so that if and when my verdict included a recommendation for surgery she would accept it without a great deal of hesitation. I knew there was going to be lots of hand wringing, eye wiping, and sniffy comments about how precious he was when the scalpel was mentioned.

When I got down to the real reason for my being there, I found that his urinary tract was blocked with a stone, called a calculus, about the size of a pea. After a great deal of palpation, I released Sir Alfred, took a deep breath of air, and started to talk.

"Mrs. V., Sir Alfred is going to need surgery," I commenced. "You probably already know that he hasn't passed any water in more than a day, and his bladder is perilously close to rupturing. Unless we relieve that pressure quickly, he will die."

As I gazed into her shocked and saddened eyes, I could see tears beginning to form. In spite of her millions of dollars in net worth, and all the privileges she enjoyed, she was still just a human being, her heart breaking over a sick sheep worth about fifty dollars.

"Are there any questions you'd like to ask me?" I stated, hoping to get her real feelings on the matter.

"Just one," she sniffed, wiping both eyes with a lacy Gucci handkerchief. "Can you tell me if my Blue Cross/Blue Shield insurance will cover this surgery?"

Perhaps that's why I've never been good working with the very wealthy. Our minds just don't think along the same lines.

I explained to Mrs. Vanlandingham that Blue Cross/Blue Shield probably would not be willing to pay for Sir Alfred's surgical expenses. However, if she wanted to call the office, I told her that I was sure that they could give her a quick ruling on sheep surgery.

"But Sir Alfred is a member of the immediate family," she pleaded, "almost like my children who are in Rome for the summer."

I started to ask her what they were doing in Georgia, but I quickly caught myself.

The operation for Sir Alfred would relieve the obstruction but it would also change his personal habits and lifestyle. Delicately put, after surgery he would be wearing a pink blanket instead of a blue one and would have to look for the room that said "Ladies" rather than the one that said "Men."

I enjoy surgery, and I also enjoy doing it quickly. It has been my experience that the quicker you can get it done, the higher the success rate—assuming, of course, that it is done properly. Therefore, I was ready to get on with Sir Alfred's encounter with the scalpel, but I wanted Mrs. V. gone from the barn. I didn't need her telling me where to make my incision or how to tie surgical knots, or asking dozens of questions at the wrong time. So I put a plan into action.

"Mrs. V., I need one of your men to help me with this, please," I stated. I figured that by the time she had fetched a gardener, I would have the incision site shaved, anesthetized, and my surgical pack up and ready to go.

Four minutes later she returned with a hired man named Floyd.

"OK, Floyd, you're gonna be my assistant," I told him. "Just hold Sir Alfred right here on this bale of hay."

Floyd said nothing, but grabbed hold of the patient with his scarred-up hands.

Just as I prepared to make my incision, I put the other part of my plan into action.

"Mrs. V., I need your help. Please go to the house and boil two quarts of water for five minutes. Let it cool for three minutes, then add four tablespoons of this solution to the water." I handed her a bottle of blue disinfectant.

As she exited the stall door, I made my incision. By the time she was halfway to the house, I had the offending stone out and in the pan.

Now for the time-consuming suturing. I knew that it would take about eight to ten minutes to complete that. If I was lucky, I would be finished by the time she arrived back in the barn. I was chattering constantly, but Floyd said nothing. He just looked the other way the entire time.

It all went as planned. When she entered the stall door, I was removing my gloves.

"Well, everything looks good so far," I announced. "As you can see, we've got things working again." The pressure was being relieved nicely and the hay and straw behind Sir Alfred was soaked.

"You aren't finished, are you?" she asked. She was holding a steaming pail of water. "What should I do with this?"

"Leave it in a cool place out of direct sunlight for five days," I replied. "If it changes color, call me right away." Before she had time to puzzle over my instructions, I went on. "That's the easy part. Now you are going to have to help him through the convalescent period. Are you a good nurse?"

"Me? A nurse? Why no!" she stammered. "What do you expect me to do?"

"Sir Alfred needs to be treated twice a day with an injection and he will have to be cleaned up if he gets straw around his surgical site."

"Oh, I can't do that! I thought you would be coming by every day on your rounds. Can't you do that while you are here?"

"Certainly I can. But you understand that I'll have to charge you for a call each time I come out. That's going to run the bill up mighty high and . . ."

"Let me assure you, Doctor, that I value this little fellow more than you can imagine," she said sharply. "And don't you concern yourself about whether I possess adequate funds to pay your fee or not. If you have any concerns, I will be glad to have the manager of one of my banks contact you about my credit rating."

"Oh no, I'm not worried about that." Now I was the one doing the stammering. She had confused me earlier in the day when she had wanted Blue Cross/Blue Shield to handle the surgical fee.

I made numerous trips to check on Sir Alfred and had many phone conversations with Mrs. V. about him. At first she called every time he ate, answered any call of nature, and even once when he sneezed. The calls the first few postsurgical days were a bit much. Actually, I considered leaving the county at one point to get away from the constant ringing of the phone.

Sir Alfred survived nicely, but I almost didn't. Mrs. V. sent a check promptly when she received our statement and even enclosed a nice thank-you note signed with Sir Alfred's hoofprint. I felt very happy, in spite of losing a couple of more years off my expected life span from such an exhausting experience.

Sir Alfred eventually succumbed to acute bloat one Sunday night while Mrs. Vanlandingham was on a cruise around the world. He discovered a fifty-pound sack of Purina dry dog food and his common sense was no match for his gluttony. Although his on-duty sheep sitter had only run to the Dairy Queen for a burger, shake, and fries, Sir Alfred had expired by the time she returned.

Unfortunately, I was the one who had to make the land-to-ship phone call to Mrs. V., who was somewhere in the Caribbean. She did not take the bad news well at all and spent a lot of time blaming herself for the tragedy.

It also fell my lot to act as funeral director. When the grieving lady returned home some weeks later, she was happy to see a beautiful, well-manicured grave complete with a pine marker. There was a carving of a little lamb on it and a short poem.

Some of my large animal veterinarian colleagues and farmer friends will scoff at the notion of pet sheep, hogs that live in the kitchen, or companion steers. Before they laugh too loud, though, they should understand that it is not our place to dictate to people what type of pets they should keep. As the number of real working farms decreases year after year, it may be that the salvation of veterinarians who prefer large animal work may rest with nonfarmer clients keeping a few cows, hogs, or sheep as companions. Often, such patients allow us to use our skills without the restraint of economic considerations.

Chapter 26

ACCORDING TO THE Choctaw County Chamber of Commerce brochures, the local weather is just wonderful, with "moderate" temperatures, "gentle" occasional rains, and "sun-filled" days. Harsh winter conditions as experienced up North are unheard-of in this "near Eden."

The brochure writer was *partially* correct. The winters aren't nearly as severe in Butler, Alabama, as are those in International Falls, Minnesota, for instance, but that doesn't mean they're easy.

I often wondered out loud if the frozen precipitation of the North would be easier to deal with than the frequent thirty-five- to forty-degree rain and constant high humidity of the South. One week would be warm, then the next would be ushered in by cold rain and sleet. You never knew what would be next. Two days before I had been over on Scott's Mountain treating a downer cow.

"Where you goin' from here, Doc?" Mr. Scott asked. He was a tough old guy, self-sufficient, set in his ways, tight with a dollar, and full of down-to-earth wisdom. I knew that in no time we would be great friends.

"Think I'll go by the barber shop and get Chappell to shear this hair off my head," I said as I plucked at the long curly stuff beginning to tickle my ears.

"No, no, Doc!" he shrieked. "It's not late enough in the winter for you to get a haircut. You'll get a cold, take pneumonia, and die!"

"Aw, Mr. Scott, people down there in town been gettin' haircuts all winter," I countered.

"Yessir, but those are town people who work inside," he allowed, "and if they go out in the cold they always wear some kind of head covering. You listen to me, Doc, we can't have you gettin' sick on us!"

When I sat down in Chappell's chair he also said something that I should have considered.

"You sure you want all this head of curly hair cut off, Doc?" he asked as he popped the striped apron out in front of me and pinned the ends of it around my neck. "It's still wintertime, you know. You might take cold and get pneumonia!"

"Chappell, I'll swear!" I bellowed. "Cut it off! Cut it off short!" The thought did run through my mind that if the barber said for me not to get a haircut, I should have listened. But I didn't.

The next afternoon a cold front, accompanied by a punishing rain, moved slowly through the area. We were trying to vaccinate a group of feeder steers at a farm in the northern part of the county when my sweat-soaked tee shirt gradually turned to a sheet of ice. By the time we had finished with the vaccinations and implants, ice had also formed on my new hairdo.

That night I started sneezing and having chills. Now I was sore all over, had a raw throat, tight chest, and earache.

"John, you've got a high fever," Jan pronounced as she felt my forehead with the back of her hand. She immediately reached for the thermometer.

"I knew that you were coming down with something when you turned down seconds on ice cream last night. Open your mouth!"

"You've got a hundred and three degrees of fever!" she exclaimed a few minutes later. "I'm calling the doctor!"

"Naw, now wait a minute," I begged. "I'm treating it myself."

"What with? Bull medicine?" she snorted.

"Well, I found some dog tetracycline capsules in the back of the truck and I'm taking those. Also I've got this big two-hundred-forty-grain cow aspirin bolus here in my pocket and I just bite off a chunk of it whenever my head gets to hurtin' real bad. It's pretty much all the same medicine anyway!"

"Of all the stupid, jackass things I've ever heard of!" she ranted. "Why do you insist on quacking on yourself instead of going to the doctor for a proper diagnosis and treatment?"

"I don't have the time to go sit all day waiting with a bunch of sick people," I answered. "I've got cows and people depending on me. Besides, he'd just prescribe the same stuff I've got in the truck, tell me to get some rest and come back next week. But I will go if I get to feeling bad enough."

"I just don't understand," she said. "You complain about farmers who think they can doctor their own cows, but then you turn right around and do the same thing to yourself."

I had been sick once before in the past five years. I was on my internship when I accidentally injected my left hand with brucellosis vaccine.

An Angus heifer had bolted through the squeeze chute at about forty miles per hour and I was too slow on the head gate. The two cowboys quickly and gleefully leapfrogged onto their sweaty horses and gave chase. After a great show of whooping and hollering, they finally cornered the reluctant beast in a briar patch and were practicing throwing their ropes at her.

I was enjoying the rodeo instead of watching where I was sticking the needle as I mixed up a new batch of vaccine. Thinking I was jabbing it into the vial of vaccine, I instead sunk the one-inch needle into the soft tissue between thumb and forefinger on my left. It buried up to the hub.

"OWWWW!" I yelled, among other things, as I quickly extracted the eighteen-gauge monster from my hand. Severe pain was working its way up to my wrist as I danced around grimacing profusely and slinging the injured extremity.

"Shoot! My hand is really boogered up now," I remember saying out loud. I applied mouth suction to the bleeding needle hole, trying to remove the vaccine. That just made it hurt. Finally, I found a teat cannula and tried infusing some penicillin. That made it hurt even worse.

"Lookie yonder, podnuh," giggled cowboy number one. "Doc's done jobbed hissef with that big o' needle!"

"Aw man, I bet t'at smarts," snickered cowboy number two. "You hurtin' too bad to fool with this calf, Doc?"

Now I was not only hurting but I was also mad. I was mad at myself for doing such a dumb thing, mad at the dumb calf, and mad at both the dumb cowboys for laughing at me. Funny how it's always guffaw time when the vet gets hurt.

"Run that sucker through the chute again and I'll show you," I fumed through gritted teeth.

This time I guillotined the streaking calf with one hand, catching her right in front of the shoulders. I kind of felt sorry for the calf when I heartily jabbed her in the neck, and I fully understood now why she bleated and struggled with such intensity.

A day later the throbbing hand had swelled to the size and consistency of a ripe cantaloupe. I could get relief only by placing it on top of my head and holding it there very still. When I started running a high fever and speaking in unknown tongues a few days later, the doctor prescribed Terramycin, aspirin, and rest. He also ordered me to come back in a week. I lost ten pounds and a lot of sleep because of the infection but I didn't miss a single call. I did not report the unauthorized human injection with Bang's vaccine to the state veterinarian's office for fear that he might require me to be tattooed, ear-tagged, or perhaps even "B" branded on the jaw.

So now I was down with some mysterious ailment probably brought on by the crazy Alabama winter weather. Sometime later Dr. Paul, our neighborhood doctor, woke me up as he stomped up to bedside. "Jan told me what you did, fool," he boomed. "Here you are, a grown, supposedly educated man, and you go get a short haircut in the winter. Then you go out in the freezing rain without a hat, and take a cold and pneumonia." He was stethoscoping my chest as he fussed.

"I haven't got pneumonia, I just . . ." I croaked.

"You sure do, boy! I'd throw you in the hospital but it's full of other people who didn't take care of themselves either. Now you just stay in this bed for a week and . . ."

"A week! A week!" I hoarsely yelled as I bolted upright. "I might lay here till dinnertime, but then I'm gettin' up from here and goin' to work. Besides, tomorrow's sale barn day! Look, just give me a shot of whatever you've got in that bag and you can be on your way to put all that money you make in the bank."

I thought I saw steam or smoke curling from his ears as he slammed shut his bag and exited the sickroom.

"Such a fine wife and kids to have to stay in the same house with such a thickhead," I heard him mumble as he marched down the hall.

Later, I had to apologize about the bank remark and ask him nicely to put a healing on my very sick system. After a month or so I was almost good as new except for losing ten pounds and some pride. Veterinarians and farmers are a whole lot alike. Neither can take the time to be sick.

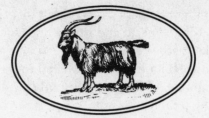

Chapter 27

WE HAD BEEN in the county for four months and the way the populace had quickly accepted us as members of the community was gratifying. We were really getting involved in civic activities. Already Jan was enthusiastically involved in the Civiettes, a women's organization that sponsored community improvement projects. She had recently chaired the highly successful annual Mothers' March for the March of Dimes.

I was a member of the county Cattlemen's Association and the Chamber of Commerce. Together we were active in the Methodist Church and the Cotillion Dance Club, and we had joined the small country club, primarily for the purpose of playing golf.

One of my classmates had taught me the basics of golf while we were in our last year of vet school, and with the used set of clubs that Jan found, I tried to play when I could find the time. At the barbershop, I met Loren Caudle, the pharmacist, and when he learned of my interest in golf, he invited me to play with his group one Sunday when they needed a fourth. After that I was hooked.

The golf course was open year round, and the true hard-core golfers played regularly, except for the occasional cold spell that made hitting the ball the equivalent of hitting rocks with a poker. But along about March, when the great weather arrived, I started playing on a regular weekly basis.

Many of my farmer clients aren't too impressed with the game of golf. First, they have the impression that it is sort of a wimpish sport played only by highfalutin country club types and that no self-respecting farmer or veterinarian would indulge in such activity.

"Golf? You mean cow pasture pool?" Stink Clark once said.

"That's the stupidest waste of time I ever heard of! Why would any-body enjoy knockin' a little white ball way down in a field, then scootin' off down there in a silly little cart to hunt for it?"

Then there's the matter of time. Golf does take a lot of daylight time since it can't be played at night. But some of my friends who would say that playing golf is a waste of time are the same ones who think nothing of spending several hours a week down at the feed store telling lies about nearly everything while sipping on cold soda waters.

Playing golf helps me to relax and lets my mind think about some-thing besides veterinary matters temporarily. Of course, some of my clients expect me to have nothing on my mind twenty-four hours a day but cat, cow, dog, horse, and sheep disorders.

Stink seemed to be worried that if I was out playing golf, I wouldn't be around to answer his emergency phone call. "Just what am I sup-posed to do if I have a cow in labor or one of my best deer dogs has a spell—drive out on the fairways and find you?" he asked.

"Why not?" I replied. "Everybody else does!" Actually, everybody didn't; but two had, and both incidents had taken place in the same month.

The first golf course interruption happened on a Sunday afternoon when we had just hit our tee shots on the first hole and were trudging down the fairway. Suddenly, I heard a car roaring down the road to the clubhouse. The horn was blowing in short, then long bursts, almost as if the driver were attempting to send out a frantic Morse code message.

We stopped and looked curiously toward the sound of the commo-tion just in time to see a Jeep-type vehicle jump the parking lot curb, cross the practice tee, and head directly in our direction.

"Lord help us!" cried Loren. "It's Penelope Carter. You better hide, John!"

"No, not Penelope!" I muttered. Quickly I scanned the area, look-ing for a place to hide. A quick escape to the sand trap, the woods, or the creek was out of the question because they were all too far away. Besides, it was obvious that she was after the veterinarian and that she had already spotted him.

"Y'all go ahead without me," I reluctantly told my fellow golfers. "I'll catch up with you a little later!" They quickly took off down the fairway.

Penelope Carter could best be described, diplomatically, as a worry wart. To her credit, she was a pet lover, animal rights advocate, and Humane Society devotee, but since I was her new veterinarian she worried the fire out of me. It was always something! She might be frantically calling about a stray cat stranded up a tree or an aged pigeon that had been chewed on by the dog or even a pastured horse she had seen somewhere along the road that looked a tad thin to her eyes.

I admired her concern for animals of all shapes and sizes, but I wished she did not have to call me multiple times a day or stop by for many private consultations. She expected me to treat all those injured strays free of charge, as well as to demand that owners of thin farm animals feed them better. It was obvious that she had not spent much time actually dealing with farmers.

"Oh, Doctor, Doctor," she panted. "Jan said you'd be just starting. Thank heavens I found you!"

"Somethin' wrong, Penny?" I asked. "You're not really supposed to drive out here in your car, you know."

"Oh, but it's Bear! He's nauseated and clawing at his mouth! See!" With that she produced a ten-pound rat terrier dog from the floorboard. He was slobbering and pawing his cheeks.

I had treated Bear before. He wasn't really mean; he just wanted to bite anybody who came within three feet.

"Been feeding him any chicken bones? Maybe he's got a chicken bone hung up in his mouth." I couldn't believe I was saying such a thing.

"No, of course not!"

"Well, let's drive over to the edge of the fairway so that impatient crowd back on the tee can play through."

Soon I was trying to examine the patient. I grabbed him by the nape of the neck and he immediately commenced writhing and wailing as loud as possible. People trying to putt on the first and ninth greens were angrily backing away from their balls and shooting angry glances in our direction.

Luckily, I saw the cause of the problem. There was a small twig tightly wedged crossways between Bear's upper teeth. I could see it easily if I pinched his neck real hard and he opened his mouth wide to yell. But how could I get the stick dislodged without sticking my finger in there and getting it bitten off?

Suddenly, I had a great idea! I went to my golf bag and retrieved my putter. I carefully eased the blade in between his front teeth so that I could wedge open his jaws and retrieve the twig with my fingers. But he chomped down on the putter with a fury.

"Oh, oh, please don't hurt him! I love him so much! Oh please!" Penelope was crying, wringing her hands, and stomping her feet, while I wrestled with the precious canine on the hood of her Jeep.

"Naw you don't, Penny!" I growled. "Nobody could love something this mean! You should have named him Satan instead of Bear!" My temper was getting out of hand now, because the little rascal was trying to scar up my favorite putter with his teeth.

By that time the golfers off the tee were arriving and were watching the show with much interest.

"Look, Buddy," exclaimed one, "that feist dog's got a putter hung up backwards in his throat!"

"Why don't you feed him dog food, Penelope?" asked another.

Penelope looked at them in disgust. "He ain't no feist! He's nearly full blood!"

"Let go of my golf club, you little sapsucker!" I growled, using one of my father's favorite words. The term "sapsucker" is about as strong a word as he ever used. If he called something or somebody a sapsucker, then they were pretty rotten and worthy of future avoidance.

About that time Bear opened his mouth to yell a little louder, so I quickly gouged at the stick with my forefinger and it popped out onto the grassy sod.

"Been feeding him wood, huh?" I said.

"I don't know where that nasty thing came from," she replied, aghast. "You know I'd never feed one of my dogs anything but the finest foods available!" She grabbed Bear and smothered him with kisses and baby talk.

"Now *I'm* nauseated," I grumbled, looking the other way.

"How's that, Doctor?"

"Oh nothing." I was just thinking about how slobbery and marked-up my putter was now. I hoped it wouldn't mess up my golf game.

"Thank you so much, Doctor. I don't owe you anything, do I?"

"Well, I . . ."

"By the way, could you come and speak at our Humane Society meeting in Meridian next Sunday afternoon?" she asked. "We meet from one to six."

"I'm sorry, I'll be playing golf."

"Well surely you can spare one afternoon to help pets! After all, you earn your livelihood from them!"

"I'll think about it. But right now you've got to get this Jeep off the golf course and I've got to join my group."

We both left in a huff. Of course, I was glad I could relieve her pet's suffering, but I was embarrassed that one of my clients would have the gall to drive a car across a manicured tee box and out on the fairway.

Well, at least no one else I knew would have that much nerve! But just two weeks later that belief would prove to be erroneous.

This time I was on the second green, bent over in deep concentration, trying to putt out, when I heard a rattletrap noise coming from toward the teebox. I looked up to see my playing partners staring openmouthed, as an apparently driverless early 1940s model red International pickup came wobbling down the fairway. It was spitting, hissing, and missing. Gray smoke was belching from its underside.

"It's Wild Eddy Neely!" said Loren. "And he's drunk, as usual."

Wild Eddy was about five feet four inches tall, and since the driver's seat springs on his truck had been defunct since before the Korean War, you could barely see the top of his bald head through the steering wheel. He was widely known for his poor driving, as well as for being one of the biggest drunks in the county. On this occasion his dual reputation was upheld in fine fashion.

As we watched, the International rocketed crazily into the rough, flattened the 150-yard marker, then plunged in amongst some small pine trees and straddled several before lurching back into the fairway.

Irate golfers were angrily pointing fingers, shaking fists, and waving number-two irons at the intruder. But Wild Eddy was oblivious to all of that.

As the truck continued its merciless onslaught on the golf course, we stood as if frozen on the green. Suddenly the truck veered again and headed straight for us. Wild Eddy was now almost standing in the seat; he seemed to be zeroing in on his favorite veterinarian. He propelled the truck wildly through the new sand trap, totaling a rake in the process, before rumbling up onto the green and skidding to a stop on the beautifully manicured putting surface. The vehicle continued to shake, rattle, and sputter for several seconds after its landing.

Taking in the scene as if hypnotized, we saw Wild Eddy creak open the door and try to climb out. Unfortunately, his right foot became entangled in a mass of baler twine on the floorboard and he dove, head first, into the soft surface of the green. His face plowed up a generous divot as he finally skidded to a stop about "gimme" putt distance from the pin.

Slowly he got to his feet. "Doc, I need ye raht now!" he slurred. It was difficult for him to stand and talk all at the same time. Drunk as he was, he was obviously upset about something.

"Will it be OK if I putt out first?" I queried, two-thirds perplexed by now. I lose patience with drunks in a hurry.

"Well, make haste, Doc, it's my cow," he said, almost in tears. "She's feelin' poorly!"

As my golfing buddies snickered and giggled, I carefully lined up my putt as Wild Eddy tended the pin. Just as I started my backstroke, he hiccupped loudly, causing me to jerk the ball off line and miss the putt by a mile. Snickering then turned into cheek-popping giggles as I neared the boiling point.

"The nerve of this drunk jerk!" I thought to myself. "I don't ask for much, just a couple of hours off every now and then to relax and play a little golf or go deer hunting. But no! Here I am, trying to get some exercise, be with my friends, and get rid of some stress, but I can't even do that."

I stomped off the green, threw my clubs into the back of his truck, and got in. As he made his return trip to the clubhouse and parking lot, his driving was as erratic as before. He ran over the greens committee chairman's golf ball, then hung our favorite magnolia tree on his rear bumper. I held my head down in shame.

"What in the world's wrong, Eddy?" I uttered through clenched teeth, just as he ran two golf carts off the cart path. I was sure I'd be ridden out of the club on a three wood.

"Doc, Little Bessie's down and can't get up and I'm awfully worried about her." He was crying by now. We lurched to a stop in the parking lot.

"OK, I'll come right over," I sighed.

"I just don't know what I'd do if Little Bess was to die," he sobbed. "She's like a member of the family. She was Eddy Junior's calf, you know, and she means so much to me and his momma since he got killed over at the state line." He wiped his eyes with a sleeve.

Once again, I thought, I shouldn't have been so quick to lose my temper. Here was a man who was deeply troubled by the loss of a son, and maybe other reasons for all I knew, and he had asked me for help. And I had gotten all riled up because he had interrupted a silly golf game.

Part of my job as a veterinarian was to help people as well as the animal kingdom, was it not? If Wild Eddy chose to drown his troubles with alcohol and act a fool, was that really any of my concern? For that matter, Penelope Carter had shown that drunks had no monopoly on foolish behavior on the golf course.

I did treat Little Bessie, and she did survive her calving paralysis problem. Wild Eddy did not do so well. Mourning the loss of his son and his excessive consumption of alcohol eventually took its toll on his body.

As for Penelope Carter, I had to write her a strongly worded letter insisting that on future visits to the golf course, she and Bear should check in at the pro shop and get assistance before Jeeping out onto the links.

As I feared, the members of the golf club were hard on me following these incidents. They assigned me to the Fairway Improvement and Greens Committee.

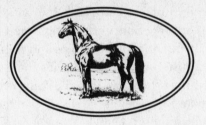

Chapter 28

THE MAIL THAT spring day brought the usual bills, junk letters informing me that I had won free vacations in Florida, checks from several clients, and the usual official State Department of Agriculture animal disease report.

But one unusual letter caught my eye. The fancy envelope was addressed to both of us and over on the back flap the embossed return address read, "The Governor's Office, Montgomery, Alabama." Below that was an imprint of the state seal.

"What in the world?" I said to myself. "Reckon what the governor wants with us? He doesn't know us from Adam!"

It was one of those envelope-inside-an-envelope deals, containing one of those little square slips of tissue paper.

"The Governor and Mrs. Wallace request the honor of your presence at the Governor's Mansion to celebrate the successful culmination of the Mothers' March fund-raiser." It also gave the date, the address, and then mentioned something about wearing a black tie.

Then I remembered Jan's chairmanship of the recent county-wide Mothers' March. They had been very successful and raised a record amount of money for the March of Dimes. That was probably what it was all about.

That afternoon when I went on farm calls, I had two things to brag about. The first was the new two-way radio in my truck. Stink Clark asked me about it.

"Doc, what's that great long fishin' pole antenna on your truck? You got a new radio?"

"Yeah boy, and it's the stuff! Now I don't have to do all that backtracking on farm calls and Jan can reach me wherever I am. Some days it saves me two or three hours of driving time," I declared.

"But don't that tall antenna hit tree limbs and things?"

"Yeah, but you've just got to remember it's there and be real careful." Later, I worked my other brag into the conversation.

"We need to palpate those heifers over across the creek, Doc," said Stink, while I was cleaning off a cow. "You got a free day in the next couple of weeks?"

"I imagine so. How about next Friday?" I asked. "No wait, that won't do. That's the day I've got to drive over to the capital and meet with the governor." I said the word "governor" kind of slow and with extra emphasis so that he would be sure to understand.

"The governor! What in the world do you want to go see him about?"

"Well, I don't particularly want to see him, but he wants to see me."

"He wants to see you! What do you reckon it is?"

"He sent this real fancy invitation, and said for me to bring Jan along," I replied. I figured it's sometimes OK to not tell the whole truth, especially in matters relating to politics.

"I can't imagine what it is." Stink was really curious now. "Were you one of those who gave a hundred dollars at the fund-raising barbecue they had for him at Rudder Hill during his campaign?"

"Naw, I wasn't living here then, remember? I was still down on the Gulf Coast," I declared.

"Boy, I'd sure like to know what this is all about," he said.

"Well, I'll let you know unless it's something secret."

I knew after I told Stink the news would be broadcast over at least half the county by sunrise the next morning. No doubt I'd be famous, at least locally. It would be in the local paper and on the radio. People would surely think that I was advising the governor on some secret political situation or a big business deal.

That night I gave Jan the letter.

"Yes, I've been wondering when the invitation was going to get here," she said. "You want to go with me?"

"Do I want to go?" I asked, shocked. "Of course! It was addressed to both of us."

"Well, that was just courtesy on Mrs. Wallace's part. You know that just the chairpersons from the sixty-seven counties are invited. Husbands may be invited but they will have no official function there at the mansion."

"OK, I'll just be your chauffeur," I said dejectedly. Boy, was that a comedown, from advisor to the governor to chauffeur in just hours.

"By the way, honey," Jan said. "Let's get the car down to Raymond Miller's and have it washed, serviced, and that transmission checked. This is very special to me and I don't want to go in a filthy car or have it break down halfway there."

"OK dear."

"Also, go by and see if you can borrow Ted's tuxedo. If you can't, then I'll have to go to Meridian and rent one."

"Why can't I just wear my blue suit? It looks fine to me."

"No, it won't do!" she exclaimed. "They'll more than likely be taking pictures sometime during the evening and I want everything to be just right. You want to look nice and professional, don't you?"

"Oh sure," I lied.

The next day I discovered that Stink had spread the news just as I had figured. About midmorning, Goat the mailman flagged me down on Indian Creek Road.

"Doc, I hear you're g-g-gonna see the g-g-governor," he stammered. "See if y-y-you can get this gravel r-r-road paved."

"I'll try, Goat, but I may not have the opportunity."

During the following days, many of my clients and acquaintances had other requests for the governor. They also advised me on what they had heard were his pet projects, his favorite football team, and other possible items that we could discuss. I was getting a lot of advice. I didn't let on to them that I was just going along as Jan's chauffeur.

"Doc, this old car's transmission is about dead," Raymond Miller told me several days later. "It's gonna go at any time."

"You think it'll make it to Montgomery and back?"

"Don't know. Might an' might not."

"You're a big help. I may be calling you to come tow me home."

"Yeah, I heard about you going over there to get the governor to pave all these old dirt roads here. Look, while you're there, make him promise to fix us a ramp to get our boats in the river over here."

On the big day, I managed to get off early and we set out for the capital about four P. M. We weren't down the road more than ten miles when the transmission started slipping while going up a long hill. After some nervous discussion, I made a decision.

"The only thing to do, Jan, is to try to get back home and just go in the truck. This car will never make another hundred miles."

At that time, pickup trucks were not afforded the same respect as they are today. It wasn't acceptable to make social visits or go to the city for dinner in an old, dirty utility vehicle. But we had no other choice. We went back and got the pickup.

"When we get there, let's park the truck down the street and walk up to the mansion. It'll just be too embarrassing for them to see us in this filthy thing."

She was right. The truck was blue and the drug box in back was white, but that was hard to tell because it was covered with red mud. The muffler had a new hole in it, which gave loud notice that I was in the area.

The seat was covered, as usual, with veterinary paraphernalia. The interior smelled of B vitamins and sheep drench. All those familiar and comfortable odors suddenly didn't seem to fit with us garbed in our best go-to-meeting finery.

Nevertheless, we made the trip without further problems or any law enforcement delay. When we arrived, however, there were no curbside parking places in front of the mansion.

"We'll have to drive up into the driveway," Jan said. "Why don't you just go up there under that little porch-looking thing and park beside those two Cadillacs?"

Two young men dressed in white shirts, black bow ties, and chauffeur's caps jumped from their posts inside a small gatehouse just as I screeched to a stop under the porch. I realized they were there to park the cars of arriving guests. However, at that point, an embarrassing thing happened.

Thong! Thong! Pow! Crash!

Suddenly the light went dim and a rain of glass showered the concrete driveway under the porch. The two attendants covered their caps with their hands and sprinted for cover. Two women in long dresses making their way up the mansion steps stopped short and looked first at us and then up at the ceiling.

I immediately knew what had happened, since I had recently

caused the same problem at the bank's new drive-in window. My long two-way radio antenna had smashed into a row of fluorescent lights on the ceiling. They make an awful racket when they explode and a worse noise when they fall to the ground.

Suddenly all was deathly quiet. All eyes were riveted on the dirty truck, now showered with shattered fluorescent light bulbs. Even the people inside the front door were pointing their fingers in our direction. The two attendants slowly and cautiously made their way back to the truck, all the while looking upward to be sure there was no more falling debris. Jan and I were both purse-lipped and silent, our lowered faces the color of beets.

"At least they don't know who we are," I said softly.

"Oh, I'm sure they'll see our Choctaw County tag and flute the news throughout the state," she said, mortified.

"Sorry about busting your lights, hoss," I said to the young man.

"Aw, don't worry about it," he said kindly, handing me a claim check. "Lots worse things have happened. A drunk judge came wheelin' in here the other night and knocked that support pillar there right out from under the roof." That made me feel a lot better.

We got out, adjusted our attire, and marched right up the steps with heads held high. I could feel the crunch of broken glass under my feet, although I couldn't hear it over the roar of my truck as it was being parked in amongst the Cadillacs and Lincolns.

The receiving line was right inside the door. There were the governor, his wife, and a bunch of other dignitaries and hangers-on.

"We're the McCormacks from Butler," Jan announced, just like we were somebody important.

"Of course, of course! Welcome!" beamed the governor, just like we were old friends. "How are things in Choctaw County? What can I help you with?" he said, pumping hands and slapping backs. I couldn't believe he actually asked the question! I was so surprised I almost couldn't answer, but then I thought of all the folks back in Butler whom I'd been bragging to.

"Actually, Governor, some of your faithful supporters did want me to see if you could use your influence to get a couple of things done over there."

"Why I'd be delighted to try. What do you need?"

"Our farmers need a road paved so they can get their products to market. Our county is just not financially able to put in a bridge and then pave it," I said. "Do you suppose the state could help?"

"Is the road named and do you know if the right-of-way is deeded to the county or state?"

"Yes, it's called Indian Creek Road and the county road grader maintains it."

"OK. What else?"

"We need a ramp built on the river so our people can get their fishing boats in and out of the water," I declared. I was beginning to get into this political stuff.

"Well, I'll be glad to look into that, first thing Monday morning." He snapped his finger over his right shoulder, signaling one of several flunkies standing behind him.

"Make a note, Billy Joe. Choctaw County. Pave Indian Creek Road. Build ramp on river. Got it?"

"Yes sir, yes sir!" The flunky was all smiles as he scribbled in a black book.

"Thank you so much, Governor. We appreciate your help," I blurted. I was still in shock.

Jan was smiling and talking about children with Lurleen Wallace. She was smiling too. Everybody was smiling.

What an evening! Soon dinner was announced and it wasn't long before Jan was receiving an award for leading her March of Dimes team to the greatest donation increase of any county in the state. She was up front shaking hands with both the governor and his wife. Several photographers were popping flashbulbs from various angles and people were clapping their hands and smiling. I was so proud of her.

Then before we knew it we were saying our goodbyes and waiting while the parking attendant brought our thundering truck around. But this time I stopped the driver before the antenna smashed into the light fixture. However, as he climbed out, a pint bottle of calcium solution rolled off the front seat and broke into a couple of hundred pieces on the street. Jan and I just got in and drove off.

Before we even got to the front gate, we were snickering about all the crazy and funny things that had happened in the past couple of hours. Snickers then became guffaws, and soon we were cracking our sides at things that wouldn't have been at all laughable under normal circumstances. Everything was funny, from a near shouting match between rabid football fans over cocktails to the look on the guy's face when the bottle of calcium shattered.

Thirty days later, Indian Creek Road was being prepared for paving. A large sign was erected stating that state tax dollars were being used, and the governor's name was displayed down at the bottom. Also, the ramp was constructed on the river in time for boating season. My friends gave me credit for getting the work done and I have never let them forget it!

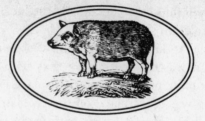

Chapter 29

MR. JIMMY THROCKMORTON was one of my best friends as well as one of my best clients. His small acreage contained a milk cow, goats, pigs, chickens, geese, turkeys, a horse, and the usual cats and yard dogs. However, his pride and joy was his pack of high-bred foxhounds. If there is such a thing as a professional fox hunter, Mr. Jimmy surely would have qualified as one. How he was able to fox hunt all night and still work hard the next day is a mystery to me.

Mr. Jimmy was tough as a gallon of nails. I often thought that he could have whacked off one of his fingers with a sorghum knife, sloshed some diesel fuel or coal oil on the stump, wrapped it up with an old fertilizer sack, and gone on about his business.

Once while he was helping a neighbor with his livestock, a 1,500-pound cow stepped on his foot, then twisted her claws around on his toes with glee. He only grimaced a little and limped around a bit for the next minute or so, but never said a word. Dog bites to hands or hammer blows on thumbs were nothing more than annoying rooster pecks. He was so tough that it was said he had once been operated on for appendicitis without the benefit of general anesthesia. They used Novocaine locally and he bit down on a dinner knife placed crossways in his mouth.

"Didn't that hurt?" someone asked.

"'Bout like bein' gored by a bull," he answered.

He enjoyed children, so after he retired from public work, he drove a school bus for the private school. When the bus had engine trouble, which was frequent, he flagged down the next passing motorist and demanded that the chairman of the bus committee be called at once.

He stayed with the children and hovered over them like a mother bantam hen.

In spite of his big heart, he took no guff from anybody. He was ready to whip a man in a minute if things got crossways. Once I actually saw him attempt to shoot a thief.

We were standing in his front yard when we heard a loud shot just up the road. Rushing to the edge of the highway, we saw a man with a shotgun throw a dead turkey into the trunk of a red Cadillac. It was one of Jimmy's turkey flock that had been relaxing the afternoon away by pecking and browsing on the road right-of-way.

"Why, that lowlife buzzard!" cried Jimmy. "He's done killed one of my turkeys! Let's go git 'im, Doc. You drive."

I was too stunned to speak, and reflexively responded to the urgency of Jimmy's order. I jumped into the driver's seat of his old Ford truck while he hopped into the other side. When I wheeled out into the road, my mouth dropped open as Jimmy retrieved an automatic shotgun from the gun rack and checked to be sure it was loaded. Then he stuck it out the window and pointed it toward the thief's car.

"Jimmy, you're not gonna use that thing, are you?" I said, still stunned.

"You just drive, Doc. I'll handle the gun," he replied. His face was the color of crimson clover in May and his mouth was set in a grim line.

By then, the unprincipled turkey assassin in the Cadillac had seen his pursuers in the rearview mirror and had liberally showered gravel, dirt, and dust all over the roadway in his urgent dash to escape. We were about two hundred yards away and momentarily gaining on the culprit.

"Jimmy, you can't—"

BLAM!! BLAM!!

The roar of the gun cut me off in midsentence. The noise also rendered me nearly deaf, setting my right ear to ringing like a cheap phone. It is amazing how loud a shotgun blast sounds in the confines of a pickup truck cab, especially when one isn't quite ready for it.

"I'll bet you anything that car's got Birmingham tags on it, too!" he roared.

That really made the crime much worse. Having one's favorite fowl slain by a "city feller" was just too much. Good down-home country folks would never stoop to anything as low-down as tame turkey homicide.

"Jimmy, hold on a—"

BLAM! BLAM! BLAM!

Then he pulled the smoking gun partway back into the cab and started rummaging through the junk on the seat, looking for more buckshot.

"Where's them blame shells?" he muttered.

The Cadillac was leaving us in a cloud of smoke. By the time I came to my senses and pulled off on the shoulder, the speeding vehicle was over the hill and out of sight. In spite of my present state of dismay, I tried to assure myself that the turkey pillager had been out of range of Jimmy's blasts.

"Whatcha doin'? Let's go! Let's go!" he shouted.

"He's long gone, Jimmy," I tried to reason. "We can't catch him in this truck. Besides, you can't go around shootin' at folks . . ."

"'Course I can! He just shot my favorite turkey!" They were all his favorites.

"Look, let's do this," I suggested. "Let's turn around and go back down to Chester's store and call the sheriff. He can notify the law up at Livingston and they can put up a roadblock there on State Highway Eleven. Then you can press charges."

"Yeah! For murder!" He was still hot, but he had started to cool down some.

We reported the dastardly crime to the authorities and they claimed they looked for the perpetrator, but without success. Jimmy always thought it was my fault that the Cadillac escaped because I didn't drive fast enough. But he consoled himself with the thought that at least one of his shots had produced bullet holes in the rear of the fleeing auto.

In spite of my shortcomings as a vigilante, Jimmy still seemed to hold me in high regard professionally. He became convinced that I was handy with a scalpel after I had performed the dental operation on his main dog, old Kate. Her facial wound had healed up beautifully, which impressed Mr. Jimmy mightily. Because of his referrals I became the veterinarian for many of the area's fox hunters.

I appreciated his confidence in my ability, but his bragging occasionally caused me some embarrassment, especially when he said that I was the best surgeon in town and he'd just as soon have Dr. John operate on him as any of 'em, and would prefer me to most. The M.D.s weren't too pleased with his endorsement.

So I was taken aback when I got a call one Monday morning from the administrator of our local hospital.

"Doc, this is Warren over at West Alabama Regional Hospital," the voice said. "Can you come over here?"

"Why sure, Warren. What's up?" I replied.

"Well, it's Mr. Jimmy Throckmorton. He's a patient here and we have him scheduled for gallbladder surgery this morning. But we can't find hide nor hair of his surgeon."

"What do you need with me?"

"Mr. Jimmy's about halfway addled with his preanesthetic injections and he says that if his doctor can't operate on him, then he'd just as soon you'd do the job." Even though Jimmy was probably hallucinating from all the sedation he'd been given, I knew he was sincere in his request.

As I motored up to the hospital, I was almost tempted to try it. After all, there's not much anatomical difference between the species. Even though the cow has four stomachs, the horse doesn't have a gallbladder, and all animals have a lot more hair or wool all over their bodies, the surgical principles are still the same. What's more, a human patient is quietly lying there snoozing soundly, offering no resistance, but barnyard animals are trying to be as uncooperative as possible, in spite of anesthesia. I always wondered if it wouldn't be a lot easier to operate on a sleeping man than on a wild, kicking bull.

Warren met me at the west wing nurses' station.

"Doc, we've got Dr. Lewis standing by to do the surgery. I need you to convince Mr. Jimmy that he's the man to do it since we can't find Dr. Perry."

"All right," I said. "Let me talk with him. With Mr. Jimmy it'll be a lot easier if you let him think I *am* doing it."

We found Jimmy lying groggily on a gurney just inside the operating room suite. He lazily opened his eyes when I squeezed his hand.

"That you, Doc?" he whispered.

"Yes Jimmy, I'm here."

"Well it's about time. Get your tools and get on with it."

I looked at Warren. He looked at me and just shrugged his shoulders.

"Nurse, let's get Mr. Throckmorton into surgery immediately!" I barked, just like I was in charge. Warren gave the nurse a nod and she wheeled the patient away.

"Where's Dr. Lewis?" I asked.

"He's on his way from radiology," someone replied. "He knows that you're here."

"I'll scrub, gown up, and go stand out of the way. Jimmy will see me there, and then you can put him under anesthesia."

The surgery took nearly two hours and it was punctuated with comparisons of human and animal anatomy.

"Your patients have gallbladder disease, Dr. McCormack?" Dr. Lewis asked.

"No," I replied. "Actually, the horse doesn't even own a gallbladder."

"Naw! I didn't know that!" he exclaimed, pausing in midstitch for several seconds while he pondered that.

He also asked me how vets were able to perform hardware disease surgery, correct displaced abomasums, and do cesarians in barnyards that were something less than aseptic.

"Just do what we have to do!" I said.

A day later, I stood by the bedside of my good friend as he talked about his surgery.

"John, I had the wildest dream," he said, slowly. "I dreamed that Doc Perry couldn't be found and you had to come in and operate on me yourself."

"Boy, that was a crazy dream," I laughed. "But you know I'm way too busy to be fooling around cutting on an old goat."

"Yeah, but I'll bet you could've done it!" he said confidently.

To my knowledge, no one ever told him that I was present in the operating room during his surgery. He is gone now, but I'm sure he always thought it was all a dream.

Most veterinarians thoroughly enjoy the profession of veterinary medicine, working with animals and their owners. We are able to perform some interesting and restorative surgery, which enables livestock to remain productive and pets to remain faithful companions longer.

It is true that we often compare our work with that of our M.D. colleagues and think about how different it would be if we never had to be concerned with the dollar value of a patient or restraint problems. How nice it would be if we always had a clean place to operate.

Make no mistake, though, most veterinarians have no desire to be in the shoes of medical doctors. They are burdened with the awesome responsibility of saving human lives every hour of the day and night. They surely deserve our respect and admiration.

Sometimes I imagine Mr. Jimmy sitting on a fluffy white cloud with other fox hunters and turkey owners. Their halos are set above their heads at a cocky angle as they swap yarns and talk about the good old days. I hope Jimmy is speaking as well of me up there as he did down here.

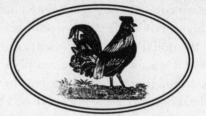

Chapter 30

As is the case with our colleagues in human medicine, probably the greatest challenge facing the practicing veterinarian, other than interacting positively with all kinds of people, is making an accurate diagnosis in each case. Whether it be an individual pet problem, a lame horse, a downer sheep, or a large herd of slow-breeding cattle, it is imperative that a correct diagnosis be made so that proper treatment can be given.

Missing a diagnosis was my greatest fear when starting out in practice. I was especially concerned about my first encounter with the most feared of all diseases, rabies. The real world symptoms of rabies frequently do not follow the textbook descriptions, and this confuses the novice veterinarian.

There are two basic syndromes, or groups of symptoms, exhibited by animals suffering from rabies. First, there is the "furious" form of rabies, where the animal exhibits extreme nervousness, belligerence, and wild behavior. Cows frequently vocalize an awful bellow, which is characteristic of the disease in that species. Since the eventual outcome in the cow is ascending paralysis and death, the victim sometimes shows odd straining movements as if trying to defecate or urinate.

Animals affected with the "dumb" form of rabies usually show no wild behavior, but instead may act somewhat depressed, frequently having hay sticking out of the sides of their mouths, because of throat paralysis. Regardless of the symptoms shown by the patient, rabies is a very difficult disease to diagnose in the live animal.

My first rabies case wasn't long in coming. I was at the sale barn one Thursday in early spring when Jan called.

"John, there's a widow woman out at Yantley who wants you to stop by this afternoon and check on a cow," she said. "They've had some rabid foxes near there, and Mrs. Pace is convinced that her old milk cow has rabies."

"What's she acting like?" I asked.

"Well, three different people have called about it and they all tell different stories. The cow is crazy as a loon, according to one of the neighbors, and the vo-ag teacher says she is slobbering all over everything and bellowing. Mrs. Pace says she just looks wild-eyed and won't eat."

"Sounds suspicious, doesn't it," I said.

As I sped toward the site of the possible rabid cow later on that afternoon, I reviewed all the possible things that looked similar to rabies. Nervous acetonemia, anaplasmosis, various plant poisonings, choke, and brain abscesses. The more diseases I mentally reviewed, the more confused I became, so I just quit thinking about that and started trying to figure out how I was going to catch the patient and examine her without getting myself exposed.

When I arrived at the small farm, it was obvious that it was the scene of unusual excitement. Several well-meaning neighbors and a few self-proclaimed cow experts were there, most sitting on or leaning upon the rail fence surrounding an apple orchard. They included a retired auction barn cowboy, the vo-ag teacher and his FFA boys there on a field trip, the soil conservation man, and the mailman. They were all huddled together in conference. Occasionally one or more of them would turn and stare intently at the patient, who could be observed quietly lying under a large apple tree. As they looked, they would rub their chins as if in deep thought, then suddenly turn back to the huddle and make some comment. The others would nod with approval.

The neighbors were mostly good citizens who worked at the paper mill and had dropped by after work to see the cow made famous by the rumor of the day.

"The veteran's here," I heard someone say, as I approached the fence.

"Naw, that must be a boy that works for him," another one said. "Nobody that young could be a real vet."

The way the experts were glaring at me, I decided to stay away from them and communicate with the friendlier neighbors, some of whom I recognized as being semipermanent fixtures at the feed mill near there. After some conversation with the group, the experts started to sidle up and make their comments.

"Young Doc," one tobacco-chewing old-timer said, "you think that t'are cow's got the hydrophobie?" Very few people called it rabies. It was either hydrophobie, rabbis, or the victim was just referred to as being "mad."

"Luke, he ain't even examined her yet!" another one said.

I decided that I had put it off as long as I could, so I carefully climbed over the fence and started gingerly stepping toward the cow lying with her rear toward me, less than fifty feet away. I made sure I had a plan of escape in case she was as vicious as some had said.

I picked up a long stick, crept up a little closer to the cow, and jabbed at her from a safe distance. The crowd was egging me on.

"Make 'er git up, young Doc! Jab 'er agin!"

"She ain't gon' do nuthin'," allowed the cowboy. "Slap 'er on the rump!"

A second poke with the stick resulted in the cow arising with little difficulty. I remember that she turned her head from twenty feet away and seemed to be examining my socks. She had some grass hanging from her mouth, like the other rabid cow I had seen, and she had that "dumb" look. While I watched, she exhibited the straining motion twice in just ten seconds, then bellowed.

"She's got the rabies, I'm sure," I announced, suddenly feeling very confident. "I think we should get her to the barn and put her in a strong stall, because she may go berserk before she dies. I'll need some help."

The crowd immediately jumped backward from the fence like it had suddenly been charged with electricity.

"I ain't *about* to get in nare with that mad cow," exclaimed nearly all the spectators, in unison.

Finally I was able to prevail upon the community spirit of the vo-ag teacher, and he helped me drive the cow to the barn.

"I'll be back to check on her tomorrow," I declared. "In the meantime, y'all leave this cow alone and don't even think about touching her."

Twenty-four hours later, I returned to the scene. Mrs. Pace and her half-sister were the only people there.

"How's the cow?" I asked.

"Aw, she's going to be just fine," she said happily. "We got an older doctor to come this morning and he said she just needed some glucose."

"Who? What older doctor?" I inquired.

"Carney Sam Jenkins!" Mrs. Pace replied. "He said he's seen a lot of cows just like this before and sometimes it was easy for young, inexperienced people to mistake low blood sugar for rabies."

I should have known that Carney Sam Jenkins would be involved in the case. After all, he lived nearby and had been *the* health expert in the area for years and years. Many folks in the immediate area wouldn't make any important decisions, especially those dealing with livestock or crops, without seeking Carney's counsel. I realized I should have consulted with him about the case.

"Did he give her a bottle of medicine in the vein?" I asked.

"No, by mouth," she answered. "And he also examined her better than you did. He checked all her teeth, her tongue, and even her tonsils!"

Sure enough, when I looked at the cow she appeared to be different from before. She still didn't appear to be eating, though.

I left in a hurry, puzzled and confused over my apparent mistake. I was just positive that cow had rabies the day before. But I was reluctant to dispute the diagnostic ability of my older, more experienced veterinary colleague.

Early the next morning I saw Carney Sam at Miss Ruby McCord's general store. I immediately asked him about the rabies suspect.

"Aw, I think she's just got nervous ketosis," he said matter-of-factly. "Didn't you smell that sweet, oniony breath? Her stomach wasn't working either."

"What about her straining? The book says . . ."

"Aw, John, a lot of that book stuff was written up North and it doesn't apply down here," he snapped. "I've seen a lot of rabid cows in this area, and she don't fit the picture. Don't be too quick to diagnose something unusual." I drove off, feeling incompetent and stupid.

Later on that week, I was busy vaccinating a drove of pigs against cholera and feeling pretty depressed about my youthful inexperience when the farmer's wife came running out to the barn.

"Dr. McCormack, you've got a phone call," she puffed. "There's an emergency. Something about a cow with rabies over at the widow Pace's!"

"I knew it!" I thought to myself. "That cow has gone berserk, broke out of the pasture, and has gored the mules and Mrs. Pace. Now she's running wild in the community." All sorts of disasters ran through my mind. The phone call was from Carney Sam.

"Doc, that cow died yesterday, and I'm sorry I didn't let you know about it then. But then I got to thinkin' about it and decided to get her brain checked out," Carney said, quietly. I could detect a moderate degree of uneasiness in his voice. "They took her over to the lab and she was positive for rabies. Now I've got to take those shots and I want you to go by the health department and pick up the serum. I've made arrangements to have my niece give me the injections. She's a nurse, you know."

When word of the confirmed diagnosis reached the community, our phone started ringing constantly.

"I touched that cow, Doc, while we were driving her to the barn," the vo-ag teacher said nervously. "Reckon I ought to take those shots in the stomach?"

"We ate some apples from those trees last fall," someone else said. "You reckon that cow slobbered on those apples back then?"

"We don't want to go mad!" someone else said.

"I bought some hay and it was cut off the pasture where that crazy cow died," another caller related. "Do you reckon my horses will die if I feed them that hay?"

The panicky calls continued for several days, each one more bizarre than the one before. The pets and livestock in the community were scrutinized more closely than ever and at the slightest hint of unusual behavior, a call to the vet was made, regardless of the time of day or night. We vaccinated many dogs, and some people even wanted their cows injected.

Putting an ungloved hand into the mouth of a rabies suspect is the one thing my professors taught me never to do. I didn't understand why Carney Sam did such a thing unless he was certain the cow had some other ailment. Several days later I saw him at Miss Ruby's store and asked him.

"Doc, I had seen a cow the night before that was choked on a small ear of corn, and I thought Mrs. Pace's cow had the same problem. I apologize for gettin' on you about makin' a quick diagnosis. I was the one who made the mistake of not lookin'."

"That's OK, Carney. The only folks who never miss a diagnosis are those who never try to make one," I replied.

I could feel our relationship growing stronger each month, even though I knew that we would still occasionally rankle each other over missed diagnoses or differences in treatment philosophies.

Carney Sam never forgot the rabies case. After that, he referred a lot of his cases my way, especially the ones that were acting furious or dumb.

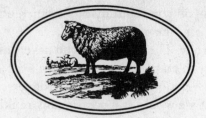

Chapter 31

"THE RODEO WILL be held on Friday and Saturday nights," the rodeo chairman announced. "And don't forget the big parade on Friday afternoon at four. All of y'all be sure to bring your horses and the entire family. We want a big turnout!"

The Choctaw County Cattlemen's Association sponsors an annual rodeo, usually held in late spring. It is a nice fund-raiser because everybody in the area attends. In the past, the only legitimate reason for missing the big event was to have a notarized written excuse from one of the county's fine doctors. You have to get it the day before, because the doctors attend the rodeo to administer first aid to the participants who have been stomped, trampled, or gored.

"Dr. John, can you ride a horse?" the chairman continued.

"Why do you ask?" I replied.

"Because we want you to be the grand marshal this year," he said.

"Me? Grand marshal? I don't know—I'm very honored, but I don't even own a horse."

"Well, you coulda rode mine," drawled Bubba Donnelly, "but it died after you doctored on it last week!" Every soul there burst out laughing.

The chuckles echoed through the meeting room for several seconds. Actually it wasn't a meeting room at all; we just met in our usual place, over in one corner of Garvis Allen's cafe. It didn't bother us not having any privacy, but occasionally strangers stopping in for an evening meal were shocked at the goings-on during our meetings.

Consider, for example, a man and his family forking into their meat loaf, cornbread, and turnip greens only to glance up and see a picture of cow worms or green medicine being drenched into a bellowing cow's mouth.

"You can borrow old Maude, Chappell's mare," someone volunteered.

"Good, that's settled," the chairman declared. "We'll start at the football field, go down by the Davis Chiropractic Clinic, then turn left and go by Harry Moore's tooth dentist office, up by Doggett Hardware, go left at the Choctaw Bank, around the square, then down by the post office to the starting point. Does that sound OK, Doc?"

"Oh sure. Just fine," I answered. But I was thinking about riding a strange horse and wondering if I could stay on her back for the entire parade. "I'll go by the barbershop tomorrow and ask Chappell about Maude."

Somehow I've never been real keen on horsemanship and hanging around with the equine set. Perhaps it's due to the fact that my youthful association with mules in those Tennessee cotton and corn fields was usually unharmonious. Another thing is that I am afraid of high places, and being precariously perched on the back of a sixteen-hand equine is farther away from the ground than I prefer to be.

Nevertheless, the next day I stopped by Chappell's barbershop to see if I could borrow Maude for the parade. Chappell was at his usual post behind the third chair. Myatt was shaving somebody I didn't recognize in the second chair, and the first chair was unattended.

"How 'bout it, Doc?" exclaimed Myatt. "What chu been cuttin' on today?"

"Nothing yet," I replied. "But you're fixin' to cut that feller there if you don't quit shakin' so bad."

I noticed his recumbent client's legs suddenly stiffen and his hands quickly clutch the arms of the chair in a white-knuckled death grip.

"Chappell, can I borrow Maude?" I yelled. I had learned to always talk loud because of his hearing.

"Borrow what?"

"Maude! Your old mare!" I hollered.

"Why sure! Just get some of that Omelene out of the crib and bang the can on the gate. She'll come up when she hears that bangin'. You gonna ride in the parade Friday?"

"Yep, I'm the grand marshal!" I proudly stated.

"Lord help 'em!" exclaimed Myatt. "With Doc in charge the whole crowd'll probably get lost and wind up in Mississippi!" All waiting for haircuts chuckled except for Myatt's customer, who still maintained his white-knuckled grip on the chair.

"Thanks, Chappell," I allowed, reaching for the door and glaring at Myatt with my best frown of disgust.

As the door slammed behind me I thought I heard Chappell's voice calling out something like "Owe you." At the time I didn't get the significance.

About midafternoon on the day of the parade, I drove the mile out Riderwood Road to Chappell's barn. I caught the mare just like he had suggested, saddled her up, and was soon cantering toward town.

"Heck, this isn't too bad," I thought to myself. "This feels pretty good sitting up this high, looking down on everybody. As long as I don't move or turn aloose of this saddle horn I'll be just fine."

My newly found riding confidence was suddenly dampened when we arrived at the Butler Creek bridge. Maude's canter slowed to a walk, then she stopped short about six feet from the little steel plate that separates road from bridge. She just stood there, looking down, her head held at an angle while she apparently contemplated the "booger" that was causing her great confusion. I dismounted, spoke a few words of encouragement into the area of her nostrils, and she immediately allowed me to lead her across the bridge. When we reached the other side, I climbed back into the saddle and enjoyed an uneventful ride on up to the football field.

The balking episode concerned me because it would prove quite embarrassing if she did the same thing when we circled the town square. But, I thought, there was no reason that such an incident would occur. We wouldn't have to cross any more bridges.

The area around the football field was mobbed with stock trailers, pickup trucks, horses of every description, and regular citizens disguised as cowboys. Even though I knew every person there, I recognized only about half of them due to their big hats, fancy snap-fronted shirts, and boots which made them walk with peculiar stilted gaits. No doubt the discount Western wear store in Meridian had done a booming business that week.

My own garb was fairly simple, including my boots. I was proudly wearing my tan Justins, which were old, scuffed, and cracked and ready for retirement. Two coats of polish and some brisk buffing had brought out a shine that made them look presentable, if not remarkable. My straw hat was a white wide-brimmed special that was in pretty good shape, having only two or three stomp scars on it and a sweat line of an inch or so around the circumference of the crown. Levi's, a white Sunday shirt, and a red string bow tie completed my ensemble.

Down at the far end of the ball field the high school band, in all their parade regalia, was practicing and getting last-minute instructions from their director. The majorettes were prancing around as if they were youthful champion Tennessee walking horses, nervous and anxious for their chance in the ring.

After fifteen minutes or so of vigorous handshaking, backslapping, boot admiring, and horse comparing, I grabbed a bullhorn out of Walter's police car and yelled.

"Let's go! Y'all follow me and the band! Let's be proud of who we are and what we do!"

Soon we were parading down the hill past the chiropractor's office, past "Bill the Pill's" cut-rate drugstore, and then down by Harry's dental office. Harry was standing out front with a bibbed patient, an elderly gentleman whose mouth was half open, obviously still very affected from Harry's Novocaine needle.

"Boy, that horse's gonna THROW YOU!" Harry yelled, laughing and pointing in my direction.

I also laughed, waved my hat to him, and continued on toward the hardware store. Then I realized what Chappell had said that day when I walked out of the barbershop!

"She may *throw you*!" Those were his exact words!

"Aw man!" I said to myself. "Now I remember! Some horse reared up and threw a boy from Yantley in this same parade two years ago. He was in the hospital for a week! I wonder if it was this horse?"

By then I was so nervous I was shaking. The distance down to the ground suddenly appeared to be much farther than before, and each hoofbeat on the concrete sounded loud and ominous. By the time we reached the town square a huge crowd of onlookers had gathered and it seemed that each set of eyes was riveted on us.

Just as I approached the Gala Theater, disaster struck. Two young lads, running around the periphery of the crowd, suddenly broke out into Maude's path. She stopped again just like she had done earlier at the Butler Creek bridge, and I lurched forward in the saddle. However, just as I went forward, one of the prankish boys dropped his minitub of popcorn and it scattered up under the mare's front end. She immediately reared up, and in doing so, the back of her head smashed into the area from the tip of my nose to the top of my forehead with a resounding *bang*!

I remember seeing a galaxy of stars and wondering if my dimestore glasses could ever be disimbedded from what used to be a pretty good nose. I don't remember falling, but I distinctly remember colliding with the pavement. Fortunately, I landed on my chest, both elbows, and the tip of my chin, in a sort of four-point landing. My thermometer case and its contents were smashed into smithereens as were the pens and other junk in my shirt pocket. I also remember laughter from the crowd and seeing the band marching in place while I gathered my wits and attempted to get back on Maude. My nose was bleeding, the front of my shirt was asphalt-stained, and everything looked real blurred since my glasses had been totaled in the crash. Of course my hat had been stomped during the accident, and it was lying there giving the appearance of a dusty pizza.

I have never been so embarrassed in my life! Fortunately, I had held on to Maude's reins and by the time I got to my feet, she appeared normal, although her nostrils were flared to the size of gallon syrup bucket lids.

Now it had become a matter of principle, pride, and determination. So in spite of, or perhaps in response to, the mirth of the crowd, I jammed a handkerchief under my nose, grimly remounted, and recommenced on my route around the courthouse, with teeth gritted.

Suddenly, I realized that I wasn't afraid of falling again. As a matter of fact, I just double-dog-dared the fool horse to throw me again. I even considered bopping her upside the head to reinforce my thinking, but thought I'd better refrain. The public frowns on horse-bopping by veterinarians.

The remainder of the parade went without problems. It appeared that those lining the streets along the final portion of the parade were unaware of my earlier problem. Apparently they thought the bloody spots on my shirt were actually red polka dots that must have been the "in" thing in Western wear.

When I returned home, Jan said nothing about the throwing episode.

"Did y'all enjoy the parade?" I asked. "I never did see you."

"Oh, yes!" she happily replied. "We planned on watching it from in front of the Gala Theater but we didn't recognize anybody there, so we went over to the opposite side of the square. I think most of the spectators on the theater side had been bussed in from Mississippi."

Of course I had to tell her about the accident when she saw my bloody shirt and asphalt-stained pants, but at least she and the kids hadn't actually seen it.

As I rested in my easy chair, I reflected that I had gotten off pretty easy. My cattlemen buddies had not been in a position to see my fall, since they were behind the band and had not yet turned the corner by the furniture store, which blocked their view. And it seemed that very few of the spectators had actually been looking at the grand marshal anyway, because they had all been staring at the beautiful majorettes.

In spite of the fall, I could take pride in being selected to lead the cattlemen's parade. Even though we had been in the county only six months, I had worked with nearly every member of the association in some kind of crisis situation—whether it was calving cows, colicky horses, or sick deer dogs. Still, proud as I was to have earned the cattlemen's approval, I made a pledge to leave the horse riding to horse people. I vowed if another grand marshal event came my way, I would ask for a red convertible sports car instead of Maude.

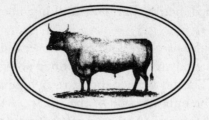

Chapter 32

"HONEY, PHONE. IT'S Miss Ruby McCord."

"Huh?"

"Are you awake, honey? You have a call," Jan repeated. Apparently, I had dozed off and was having a nightmarish time staying on that horse the second time.

"Yeah, yeah, I'm awake."

I slowly dechaired and trudged to the phone halfway down the hall. I was stiff and sore from the horse ride just hours ago.

"Hello, may I help you?"

"Yes, Doctuh. This is Ruby McCord. One of our neighborhood farmuhs has a mule that is somewhat ill," she said, properly. "From what he tells me, I fear that he may be in misery from locked bowel disease."

"Yes ma'am, I see. Is the mule in pain?" I asked.

"Just a minute, Doctuh." I could hear her quietly conversing with someone there with her.

"Oh yes, he's wallowing, pawing the earth, lying down and getting up," she replied.

"OK, now what have they already done for the animal?" I asked. I heard more mumbling and low talk.

"Doctuh, the man now says they feel like the mule has suffuhed an attack of kidney colic, so they have already tried the usual remedy of applying warm turpentine to the navel. They've done that three times in the last two hours without obtaining any appreciable relief."

It was always a treat listening to Miss Ruby talk. Her grammar was so proper and some of her pronunciations were so typically Old South they practically dripped with magnolia blossom nectar.

"The mule belongs to Mr. Kent Farris. I believe he said you had been theah befoah to treat some cows that had eaten too much cawon." Well, that was one way of putting it.

"Oh yes ma'am, I have been to his place two or three times this year. Tell him I'll be on up there in about thirty minutes. And tell him to walk that mule."

Colic is a broad term indicating abdominal pain, and it is a common malady in equines, probably because of their long and complex digestive tracts. Portions of the tract may get twisted, trapped, or simply filled with gas. Regardless of the cause or severity, equines unfortunately possess a low pain threshold and quickly exhibit signs of abdominal distress. The pain can be mild or it can be excruciating and unrelenting, depending upon whether it is caused by excessive gas or a complete blockage of some portion of the gastrointestinal tract.

"Uh, theah's one more thing, Doctuh," she said slowly. Miss Ruby seemed to be having trouble describing the rest of the animal's symptoms. "Mr. Kent is afraid the mule's kidneys are completely locked up, because he, uh, keeps trying to make watuh, but can't."

That was another common dirt-road diagnosis. Because of the pain, a colicky horse or mule frequently stands with front and rear feet far apart in a stretched-out position, as if trying to urinate. Back then, this condition was thought to be "kidney colic," although it is nothing more than the animal's attempt to get relief from the pain.

Since departing veterinary school I had noticed that mule colic seemed to be a common event in the spring of the year, and it nearly always occurred after dark.

Some of my veterinarian colleagues claim that springtime colic is due to the bot worms moving inside the stomach and causing all that discomfort. Others say that lush, green, watery clover and native grasses contain some smooth-muscle-spasming compound which acts swiftly when consumed by greedily grazing equines. Some folklore believers blame the gas and griping on evil spirits, cold creek water, the spring moon, or bad blood.

At that time many mule owners were poor, small landholders, and they always grew a few acres of cotton. Since tractor power was unaffordable except to those few individuals who worked in town, the mules provided the plow power.

My explanation for the springtime colic had to do with the change in lifestyle because of the season. All winter long the mules had lazed around in their lots and stalls and had been on minimum daily rations of a couple of ears of corn and a flake or two of grass hay. When plowing time came in March or April, they were suddenly called upon for a day's work. They responded by pulling the plow with enthusiasm, especially if pointed in the direction of the barn. Their hairy coats became hot and steamy, and sweat lathered up in foamy layers where the gear and reins made intimate contact with hide.

By nightfall, both man and beast would be exhausted, yet both felt good about the honest day's work they had put in. Both quenched their thirsts from the clean creek that bordered the fields before heading for home.

In the barn, the mules were given an extra ration of corn as a reward for working so hard. But their digestive systems couldn't cope with the change in their ration. That's why, a few hours later, the gas and intestinal cramping caused the symptoms of colic, and the veterinarian was summoned.

As I motored up the road to Mr. Kent's farm, I reviewed my colic examination procedure. First, I would make an overall visual inspection of the patient at a distance, checking for signs of anxiety, depression, and general demeanor. Next, I would check gum color, pulse, heart, and respiratory rate and listen to gut sounds with my stethoscope. Finally, moving on to the rear, I would take a temperature if I thought it was possible to do so without sustaining a serious injury from flying hooves.

It was dusk when I turned into the Farris driveway, and I noticed that half the small two-acre field in front of the house had been freshly plowed. The mule-drawn plow had been left at the end of the row, ready for the mules again the next morning. I assumed that Mr. Kent would plant cotton again there, just as he had every year for the past forty years or so. Too much land in the South was like that two-acre plot—it had been "cottoned" to death.

At the barn, Mr. Kent was out front slowly walking the mule back and forth, pausing occasionally to see if the sick patient would attempt to go down. On the house side of the barn was an old International pickup truck backed up onto an embankment. It was Carney Sam Jenkins's truck, and he was sitting on the right front fender whittling on a piece of hickory with his old Boker Tree brand pocket knife. His mouth was flapping, as usual.

"Probably lecturing on kidney colic and turpentine deficiency to that bored guy standing with him," I thought. The guy was "Wormy," the runt who always seemed to be in the vicinity of Mr. Kent's farm when veterinary problems arose.

"How's it goin', y'all?" I asked. Carney Sam spoke first.

"Hey Doc, that ole mule just can't git no relief. Wants to git down and roll, and I just can't get them kidneys to unlock. I've turpentined his navel three times!" I could hear the soft clop, clop of the equine's feet on the barnyard clay as Mr. Kent came closer to the truck.

"Let Doc check 'im over, Kent," ordered Carney Sam. "Maybe he can give a shot of wonderful drug or something."

Carney had read about the wonder drugs such as penicillin and other germ-killing medicines, but he called them "wonderful" drugs. I catch myself doing the same thing occasionally.

I started my examination just as I had intended, but this time accompanied by a discourse from Carney Sam. The mule's eyes and gums appeared normal, pulse forty-eight, respiration sixteen, and heart sounded good. Carney Sam was now getting into the meat of his long-winded dissertation on equine internal medicine. I noticed that what he lacked in factual knowledge, he made up for in enthusiasm. Wormy seemed to be enjoying it, because his head was constantly nodding.

When I pulled my stethoscope from the rear pocket of my coveralls, Mr. Kent looked puzzled.

"What's that thing fer, Doc? It looks like what a real doctor listens to a feller's heart with," he allowed.

"You're right as rain, Kent," Carney Sam declared, "and he's gonna listen to that mule's belly and . . ."

Things got muffled as I placed the stethoscope head over the heart, then at various spots of the lungs and abdominal cavity. Occasionally the mule would make a halfhearted attempt to go down, but Mr. Kent would talk right stern to him and slap on his neck.

"Git up! Git up from there, Jake!" he'd yell. The startled Jake would straighten up quickly and look around at the stethoscoped figure at his side.

Finally, I removed my big thermometer from its black carrying case, slung it hard a couple of times, then quietly made a move toward Jake's rear end. But when the cold mercury of the thermometer tip made contact with the sensitive skin under Jake's tail, he suddenly double-kicked the side of the barn, narrowly missing my left knee.

Pow! Pow! The side of the rickety barn shuddered, and splinters rained down like confetti. The thermometer had flipped backwards out of my hand from the force of Jake's kick and had half-buried itself in a pile of barnyard excrement some thirty feet away.

"Did he break it, Doc?" asked Carney Sam, as I retrieved it with fingertips and wiped it on some handy straw.

"Naw, it says one-oh-two-point-three degrees. Normal is about one-oh-one-point-five," I declared, gazing intently at the mercury column and standing well out of reach of Jake's rear end. "Isn't that right, Carney?"

"Right as rain, Doc," he answered. That was one of his favorite sayings.

"You took it that quick!" exclaimed Wormy.

"Yeah, this one gets a real quick reading, 'cause it's made 'specially for jumpy mules," I lied. "This would have been a good time to just feel of his forehead," I thought to myself.

"It's his kidneys, ain't it Doc?" inquired Carney Sam, still whittling.

"Carney, I believe he's got an impacted colon and he's gassy in his small intestines. If he had kidney problems, his pulse and respiration would be a lot higher. Also, the pain he's having is a mild dull pain, not the wallowing-around-on-the-ground kind of pain. What we need to do is pass a stomach tube and pump a gallon of mineral oil into him so it will get that stuff on out of him. Then we'll give him something for the pain to see if we can't get him easy."

Carney Sam pursed his lips as if he wasn't convinced my diagnosis was correct, and I could hear him mumbling while I extracted my equipment and medicine from the truck.

"I don't know about Doc," I heard him say to Wormy and Mr. Kent. "He does real well on sick dogs and deliverin' calves, but I don't understand how he could miss something as easy to spot as the kidney colic."

I'd heard all that before and I was used to it. I could depend on my clients playing their usual game of second-guessing the vet, and Carney Sam was the area's leading expert in the field. I just smiled to myself and continued on with my work.

"Doc, if his kidneys ain't locked up, how come he keeps tryin' to make water?" asked Carney.

"Because his pain receptors tell him that there is pain somewhere behind his diaphragm area. Remember, he's never read an anatomy book like you and I have, so he doesn't know whether it's ileum, ventral colon, pancreas, kidneys, or what that's hurting. So the first thing he tries to do is stretch out like he's gonna make water and that stretching makes him feel better. Then when it gets worse, he'll wallow and roll around on the ground. But that's dangerous 'cause he's liable to get his jejunum tied up with his cecum."

As I had expected, this quieted the peanut gallery. There was silence except for the sound of Carney's clip blade making rhythmic cutting strokes on his wood. All three men, and Jake, were standing in slack-jawed confusion, pondering that strange explanation of equine belly pain. Finally, Mr. Kent pointed to the tube in my hand and spoke.

"Doc, which end of this mule are you gonna put that garden hose in?"

"Well, it's a special mule stomach tube and I'm gonna put it up his nose and down into his stomach," I declared.

"He ain't gonna like that," exclaimed Wormy.

Wormy was right. I had already found that efforts to pass nasogastric tubes in blue-nosed mules frequently resulted in severe damage to the front side of the tube manipulator's body. In addition, if the procedure was being carried out within one hundred yards of any pickup truck, a chaotic struggle often resulted which ultimately made its way to the hood and windshield of the vehicle. Therefore, passing a large rubber tube up through an equine's nose requires great skill on the part of the tuber and a little cooperation on the part of the tubee.

The tube must be kept down in the lowest portion of the nasal cavity. Most of the time it is necessary to apply a twist to the nose of the equine with a twitch, in order to divert attention from the tubing process. The twitch causes some "discomfort," as I often hear physicians pronounce just before they pull out a chest tube or something equally painful.

If the tube is kept low and eased carefully through the nose, it will soon reach the throat. At that point the tubee must perform a very basic manipulation. He must swallow when he feels the tube tickling his throat. The act of swallowing directs the tube into the esophagus, and then with a few pushes from the tuber, the tube is quickly seated in the stomach.

The trouble is, mules aren't in favor of swallowing tubes. Being a lot smarter than horses and more ornery as well, they can tell that a tube is not oats or alfalfa. So a tubed mule just tightens up his throat and refuses to swallow, which directs the tube into the windpipe. That's when the trouble starts.

No mule can stand it for very long when the tube scratches the interior of his windpipe. That's when they start walking on air, throwing their heads, stomping over truck hoods, and trying to hurt veterinarians.

Mule psychologists would probably say that the tickling tube is just an excuse for the beast to turn violent. He's already riled about being put on the earth as a mule, with nothing to ever look forward to except for old hard ears of corn and an occasional kicking fit. With all these thoughts bouncing around inside my brain, I applied the twitch to Jake's nose.

"Awright now, Mr. Kent. You've got to hold on to this twitch and stand around here on the off side while I try to work from the other side. Carney, one of y'all might ought to steady his rear end in case he starts to sashay around."

Carney slowly stood, raked the shavings from his lap, folded and pocketed his knife.

"Whoa boy, whoa now," he said softly, patting Jake on the rump. "OK Doc, go ahead."

I began to ease the swallowing end of the tube up Jake's left nostril. Surprisingly, he offered no resistance other than flaring his nostrils and tensing up a bit. I knew that he was beginning his throat-tightening action which would close off the esophagus but leave the windpipe open. It is odd how some equines know how to do that even though they've never seen a stomach tube.

The tube kept slipping into his windpipe which instantly initiated spasms of raspy mule hacks and coughs, accompanied by exaggerated head bobs and attempts to strike out at his tormentors with his front hooves. He was dragging the three men around in circles and I was becoming concerned about damaging Carney's ancient truck or some of the farm machinery scattered at random around the barnyard.

I was rubbing the mule's throat with one hand and pushing the tube to and fro with the other.

"Come on Jake, swallow the thing!" screamed Carney Sam. "Swallow, you suck-egg mule!" At that instant he delivered a swift kick to Jake's belly with his size eleven engineer's boot.

The startled Jake relaxed his throat muscles briefly and in seconds the tube slowly slid right down into the stomach. With the hard part over, I then pumped in the oil, mixed with an ounce of turpentine.

"Gonna put that whole gallon in 'im?" asked Wormy.

"Yep. And whatever you do, don't stand behind him after about three o'clock tomorrow afternoon," I declared, removing the tube. Everybody snickered, thinking about the aftereffects of such a voluminous laxative.

Seconds later I was injecting a sedative and smooth-muscle relaxant into the mule's jugular vein.

"Now let's walk him for a while and just see."

Wormy took the lead rope and started around the barn while we gathered up equipment and headed toward the well for the dreaded cleanup process. It is amazing how much mineral oil gets smeared on everything just from the remnants of a one-gallon dose. My stainless steel bucket, stomach pump, dose syringe, and eight-foot tube were all slick with the stuff, and the front of my coveralls now had assorted lardlike splotches from all the splatters and hand wipes. But some ten minutes, three drawings of well water, and a lot of green soap scrubbing later, the equipment was clean. The coveralls were Jan's department, and I knew she'd fuss a little about the stubborn oil spots that she couldn't get out.

"He's passin' gas! And a heap of it!" yelled Wormy.

"Good! Now maybe he'll get some relief," exclaimed Mr. Kent.

"Now he's passin' water! A heap of it! *Whooo weee!*" Wormy reported. Curiosity got the best of Mr. Kent, so he hurried back to the barn to see the gas- and water-passing events. I looked at Carney and he stared back at me for a few seconds before either of us spoke.

"What do you think, Carney?" I said. I thought maybe he'd be pleased about all of Jake's suddenly emptied abdominal organs, or he might possibly acknowledge the value of my modern veterinary skills. I should have known better.

"Doc, you're a smart man. You've done a lot of good since you moved in here a few months ago, and everybody in this county is mighty tickled to have you here. Now you treated this old mule here just right and it worked. But think about what just happened inside that mule."

"What do you mean?"

"Well, I think you ought to realize that he was locked up in the kidneys *and* bowels. Your medicine unlocked both organs because you put it inside the body and it worked quicker than letting the navel soak it up from the outside. That vet school talk is fine, Doc, but don't go hard against tradition and experience in Choctaw County, because we've been having kidney colic around here for years and years."

I sighed. In spite of some of our diagnostic and treatment differences, Carney and I had become good friends, and he was responsible for a lot of the calls that I had received. But every time I thought I had taught Carney a lesson about veterinary medicine, he'd say something to remind me I had a long ways to go. Fortunately, I didn't have to think of a response to his comment because just then Wormy, Mr. Kent, and Jake walked up.

"Doc, he acts fine now. He's not hurtin' and he wants to nibble on grass," declared Mr. Kent.

A quick examination revealed that Jake's heartbeat and respiratory rate were reduced somewhat and he wasn't showing the anxiety of a half hour ago.

"Why don't you turn him aloose over there in the barn lot for the night. Don't give him any feed or hay tonight. Tomorrow morning give him a flake or two of hay," I suggested.

It was almost dark when Wormy released Jake in the lot. Jake cavorted around like a young colt, jumping and kicking. It was a remarkable recovery.

"Doc, come on in the house, if you got the time. Y'all too, Carney and Ed." That was the first time I'd heard Wormy's real name.

"Can't this time, Kent," replied Carney. "Got to go feed up and then me and Ed are supposed to go fox huntin' later tonight with that Jimmy Throckmorton crowd. See ya', Doc. Remember what I said."

"Thanks for your help, Carney. Don't let that fox huntin' crowd get you in trouble with the game warden," I replied.

We made small talk walking up the hill to the house, chatting mostly about sick equines and their treatment. I thought how pleasurable it is for a veterinarian to be invited into a client's home, and it was especially gratifying for me at that time in the growth of the practice.

Mr. Kent strode briskly across the worn linoleum floor to a wooden cabinet, collected two large peanut butter glasses, and set them on the counter near the single water faucet. Then he squeaked open a door underneath the sink and brought forth a small-mouthed gallon jug half full of a transparent liquid. As Mr. Kent disturbed the solution, its surface beaded up briefly like tiny ice crystals, but quickly smoothed out when the shaking ceased.

With a ceremonious air, Mr. Kent twisted the top off and carefully poured each glass two-thirds full of his homemade moonshine liquor. It was obvious he was immensely proud of it and wanted to share it with a friend.

I knew the Law would send someone to prison for making moonshine whiskey, but I wondered if the Lord would send someone to Hell for making a product that took so much time, tender loving care, and know-how.

"Doc, there's a little taste fer ye'. See what you think about it."

While I was pondering the product and wondering what I was going to do with it, Mr. Kent grabbed a shovel from a corner and disappeared out the back door.

I continued to stare at the crystal-clear liquid. It seemed to be staring back at me. Finally, I dipped a finger into it and raked it across my tongue. It was right hot and I didn't know whether I could get even an ounce of the fiery stuff past my lips and down my throat. But if I didn't, Mr. Kent's feelings would be hurt.

I realized this might be the moment of truth for me in the community. Sort of a test of my loyalty to the homemade liquor industry or an initiation into the moonshiner's inner circle. I didn't want to be a member of that group, but I did need and want to be the first person they thought of when an animal health problem arose. I also knew that being invited into Mr. Kent's kitchen was an honor afforded to few "outsiders," and the least I could do was to show respect for his product.

I stepped quickly across the creaking floor and gripped the counter by the sink. Then I saw my reflection in the bare window as I slowly raised the eight-ounce peanut butter glass to my lips and took a small-sized quaff of Mr. Kent's finest. The face reflected in the window now appeared popeyed and a near panic-stricken look came over it, which coincided with the cauterizing effect that was taking place inside my oral cavity.

The first few seconds weren't too bad, but then the burning commenced in earnest. It was as if there were a long fuse that had been lit in my throat and it was working its way all the way down to my stomach. I remember gasping for air, then frantically coughing and trying to clear my throat of the damaged tissue that was obviously left in the wake of the draught. The facial expression in the window seemed to be that of a man who had just been informed that the IRS was on the phone demanding the keys and title to his favorite pickup truck.

Finally, the torture subsided somewhat, and I began to wonder how much internal damage had been done. I knew that if my constitution survived the burning assault, I would for sure have a healthy, worm-free gastrointestinal tract for the rest of my life.

But there was still the matter of the remaining liquor, almost a half glass of it. When I heard Mr. Kent's step on the stoop, I quickly poured most of it down the drain. I'm sure I heard a hissing sound as it cleaned out his pipes.

Seconds later, he came shuffling into the room with a half-gallon Kerr fruit jar cradled in his arms. It was full of the same clear liquid, but it was covered with mud, dirt, and grit. As Mr. Kent rinsed it off in the sink, I surmised that the stuff had been buried somewhere out back, maybe for a long time.

"Doc, was that smooth or what?"

I opened my mouth to speak, but nothing came but a hoarse whisper. I cleared my throat and made a second effort.

"Yes. It's a fine batch. Splendid," I managed to rasp out through my tormented vocal cords. I figured this would be another time I would be forgiven for lying.

"Your glass is nearly empty. Like another little taste?" I wondered what a full-fledged big taste would have done to me.

"Can't Mr. Kent, got to get on 'cause I may have another call."

"Doc, I appreciate what you did for my mule. And I want you to take this jug home with you and see what you think about it."

"Well, thanks a lot, you are mighty generous." My voice was getting better, but the fire was still burning in my belly.

Later, while driving home, I wondered what I would do with the big jug and whether or not Mr. Kent had discovered my discarded moonshine in the sink. I suspect that he had the cleanest sink pipes in the community.

A few minutes later I was walking into the house to meet a happy welcoming committee of Tom and Lisa. Both rushed my way making joyous noises, the likes of which are surely music to the ears of any proud father and remind him to make sure his priorities are in the correct order. Then Jan had some interesting news.

"Honey, a little while ago, Loren Caudle and a couple of others came by to report that you have been asked to become a member of Rudder Hill Hunting Club. I told them you'd probably have to think about it," she said, smiling.

"Yeah, for about five minutes! Wonder how that came about? I thought you had to be around here a long time before the natives would even consider you for membership."

"From what they said, Carney Sam Jenkins was the one who recommended you. I reckon he must think a lot of you, because they don't let just anybody become a member. Now you can go to all those great barbecues on organized deer-hunting days, plus meditate in the woods anytime you please while listening to the sounds of nature," she declared.

Later that night, after the kids were fast asleep and I was feeling almost normal again, Jan and I sat out on the front steps with Mickey and Go Back, thinking about all that had happened in just six short months of practice. As we stared up at the stars through the tops of the loblolly pines, Jan said to me, "Already feels like home, doesn't it?"

I realized she was right. A veterinarian becomes part of a rural community very quickly. Everybody has animals that need help, from the hired hands and dirt farmers to the Mrs. Vanlandinghams. The vet steps into their lives in an intimate way—maybe only for an hour or two, but often it's long enough to create a friendship. Not only had Choctaw Countians accepted my professional ability and provided enough income to support our family, but they had accepted us warmly as neighbors, too. Carney Sam Jenkins had even gotten me into Rudder Hill!

I guess I had made some progress with him after all.

ABOUT THE AUTHOR

Dr. JOHN MCCORMACK is a Professor of Veterinary Medicine at the University of Georgia. He lives in Athens, Georgia.

Look for the further adventures of John McCormack in *A Friend of the Flock: Tales of a Country Veterinarian* (Crown). Now available wherever books are sold. Here's an excerpt:

From *A Friend of the Flock: Tales of a Country Veterinarian*

"You've bought what?" I exclaimed, five seconds after I walked in the back door.

"A lot," Jan replied.

"A lot of what?"

"You know, a lot. A piece of land where we'll build our veterinary clinic," she declared.

"Did you pay for it?" She nodded her head affirmatively. I was so surprised that I forgot to ask where it was located.

"What with? I didn't know we had any money!"

"Well, I've been putting a few dollars aside because I knew that an opportunity like this was going to present itself soon," she replied. Either Jan's extrasensory perception is highly developed, or she has an amazing faith in the future. She is always uttering positive slogans, such as "Just be patient, things will work out" or "I've got a feeling that the time is right for this," and she is usually right.

"Now tell me about it. What happened? Why didn't you call me on the two-way?"

"I tried to, about three o'clock, but you must have been away from the truck or out of range. Speed called and said that when people had heard about the availability of the lot, they were calling and lined up wanting it. But he wanted us to have first refusal on it, so I had to make a decision right then. I just knew that you would want me to go ahead with it."

"Why was he even selling it?"

"Seems it belonged to someone out at Lisman who had planned to build a house on it, but due to some family problem they decided to build closer to home. The lot has even been graded, so there's very little site preparation necessary. Speed even told me about a reputable builder who specializes in small block buildings, if that's what you are sure you want." She was talking just like a contractor, but I was unaware that she had any previous building experience. Perhaps women are just born with the nest-building gene and it comes naturally.

I knew exactly how I wanted my clinic building to look. I had drawn the plans on notebook paper over and over while "studying" in veterinary school. It would be of simple concrete block construction, with the blocks stacked, not staggered, a flat-topped roof, and dimensions of approximately 40 feet by 20 feet. Naturally, Jan's building genes told her that a building of only 800 square feet was much too small and I would not be satisfied with such a "peewee" building. But I knew what I needed and I didn't want to waste a lot of time tromping around in a big, sprawling clinic. Besides, if I needed more space I could easily add more room later. She disagreed, of course, but we had agreed that the clinic was going to be my baby and the new house she had planned would be hers. I shuddered to think what she could do once turned loose to plan an entire house!

* * *

"Where is this land that we just bought, Jan?" I asked excitedly. Even though she had been using builders' language, I was a little concerned about her ability to walk a piece of land and envision a clinic building sitting there.

"It's about a quarter of a mile north of the courthouse, on the west side of Highway 17. It's not the best lot I've seen, but it is very convenient and the price was right."

"Let's go look at it right now, before it gets too dark."

Less than a mile and two traffic lights later, we slowly drove down the hill to where I could see a yellow streamer hanging from a sapling on the west side of the road. Stopping in the road, Jan pointed to the streamer.

"See that marker? That's the southeast corner. From there it goes north along the road nearly 400 feet, then west 200 feet alongside that small branch, then due south about 300 feet, and from there back to this starting point," she exclaimed, still pointing out the landmarks. I was surprised that she could remember each dimension with such accuracy. She was quoting figures, while I was thinking acres. That must be close to two acres, I thought to myself. But then I realized the back dropped off into a ravine, which would be useless unless filled in. Nevertheless, there was more than enough space on the level part for any structure that we would ever want or need.

As we proudly stood on the roadside gazing at our parcel purchase, vehicles occasionally passed and the smiling drivers would honk their horns, obviously aware of what was transpiring. No doubt they'd been informed by the efficient Choctaw County information bureau, otherwise known as the barbershop and beauty parlor rumor mill.